Student Study Guide to Accompany

Psychiatric Nursing: Biological & Behavioral Concepts

Second Edition

Student Study Guide to Accompany

Psychiatric Nursing: Biological & Behavioral Concepts

Second Edition

Deborah Antai-Otong, MS, APRN, BC, FAAN
Veterans Integrated Systems Network (VISN 17)
Program Manager, Care Coordination Home Telehealth
Arlington, Texas
Mental Health Provider, Ft. Worth Outpatient Mental Health Clinic

Prepared by
Peggy L. Hawkins, PhD, RN, BC, CNE
Professor
Associate Dean, Health Professions
College of St. Mary
Omaha, Nebraska

Previous edition prepared by
E. Monica Ward-Murray, RN, BSN, MA, EdM, EdD
Assistant Professor/Assistant to the Dean for Research
North Carolina Agricultural and Technical State University
Greensboro, North Carolina

THOMSON

DELMAR LEARNING

Student Study Guide to Accompany Psychiatric Nursing: Biological & Behavioral Concepts, Second Edition
By Deborah Antai-Otong, MS, APRN, BC, FAAN
Prepared by Peggy L. Hawkins, PhD, RN, BC, CNE

Vice President, Health Care Business Unit:
William Brottmiller
Editorial Director:
Matthew Kane
Acquisitions Editor, Nursing:
Maureen Rosener

Senior Product Manager:
Patricia Gaworecki
Marketing Director:
Jennifer McAvey
Marketing Channel Manager:
Michele McTighe

Marketing Coordinator:
Chelsey Iaquinta
Content Project Manager:
Jessica McNavich

ISBN-13: 978-1-4180-3875-5
ISBN-10: 1-4180-3875-X

Notice to the Reader

Publisher does not warrant or guarantee any of the products described herein or perform any independent analysis in connection with any of the product information contained herein. Publisher does not assume, and expressly disclaims, any obligation to obtain and include information other than that provided to it by the manufacturer.

The reader is expressly warned to consider and adopt all safety precautions that might be indicated by the activities described herein and to avoid all potential hazards. By following the instructions contained herein, the reader willingly assumes all risks in connection with such instructions.

The publisher makes no representations or warranties of any kind, including but not limited to, the warranties of fitness for particular purpose or merchantability, nor are any such representations implied with respect to the material set forth herein, and the publisher takes no responsibility with respect to such material. The publisher shall not be liable for any special, consequential, or exemplary damages resulting, in whole or part, from the reader's use of, or reliance upon, this material.

Contents

Preface   **vii**

UNIT 1   **PERSPECTIVES AND PRINCIPLES**   **1**

1   History of Psychiatric Nursing 3
2   Concepts of Psychiatric Care: Therapeutic Models 9
3   Interfacing Biological-Behavioral Concepts
   into Psychiatric Nursing Practice 17
4   Foundations of Psychiatric Nursing 21
5   The Nursing Process 27
6   Therapeutic Communication 31
7   Cultural and Ethnic Considerations 37
8   Legal and Ethical Considerations 41

UNIT 2   **RESPONSE TO STRESSORS ACROSS THE LIFE SPAN**   **45**

9   The Client with a Depressive Disorder 47
10   The Client with a Bipolar Disorder 53
11   The Client with an Anxiety Disorder 57
12   The Client with a Somatization Disorder 61
13   The Client with a Stress-Related Disorder 67
14   The Client with Schizophrenia and Other Psychotic Disorders 71
15   The Client with a Personality Disorder 75
16   The Client with Delirium, Dementia, Amnestic,
   and Other Cognitive Disorders 81
17   The Client with Attention-Deficit Disorder 87
18   The Client with a Dissociative Disorder 93
19   The Client at Risk of Suicidal and Self-Destructive Behaviors 97
20   The Client Exhibiting Aggression, Hostility, and Violence 103
21   The Client with a Substance-Related Disorder 107
22   The Client with an Eating Disorder 115
23   The Client with a Sleep Disorder 123
24   The Client with a Sexual Disorder 129
25   The Client Who Survives Violence 133

UNIT 3	THERAPEUTIC INTERVENTIONS	141
26	Individual Psychotherapy	143
27	Group Therapy	149
28	Familial Systems and Family Therapy	155
29	Psychopharmacologic Therapy	161
30	Electroconvulsive, Other Biological (Somatic), and Complementary Therapies	167
31	Crisis Intervention Management: The Role of Adaptation	173
32	Milieu Therapy/Hospital-Based Care	179
33	Home- and Community-Based Care	185
34	Psychosocial Care in Medical-Surgical Settings	189

UNIT 4	ADVANCING PSYCHIATRIC NURSING PRACTICE	195
35	Psychiatric Consultation-Liaison Nursing	197
36	Psychiatric Nursing Research	205
37	The Future of Psychiatric Nursing	211

| ANSWERS | | 219 |

Preface

The *Student Study Guide to Accompany Psychiatric Nursing: Biological & Behavioral Concepts,* second edition, is designed to enhance your understanding of mental health nursing. As a complement to the textbook *Psychiatric Nursing: Biological & Behavioral Concepts,* second edition, this tool will challenge you to recall and apply the facts, concepts, and principles found in the core book. Use this resource with the goal of becoming prepared and knowledgeable in the area of mental health nursing. Each chapter of the *Student Study Guide* corresponds to the material covered in the same chapter found in the *Psychiatric Nursing* textbook and includes the following:

Activities

"What are the characteristics that distinguish one disorder from another?" "Can you identify and explain treatment options for a client with a particular condition?" These types of questions are found within matching, short answer, and fill-in application exercises of the core text material. New to this edition are self-assessment questions based on case scenarios to enhance critical thinking skills. The process of completing these activities will reinforce the skills and knowledge necessary to become more comfortable with the content area and prepare you for practice.

UNIT 1

Perspectives and Principles

Chapter 1   History of Psychiatric Nursing

Chapter 2   Concepts of Psychiatric Care: Therapeutic Models

Chapter 3   Interfacing Biological-Behavioral Concepts into Psychiatric Nursing Practice

Chapter 4   Foundations of Psychiatric Nursing

Chapter 5   The Nursing Process

Chapter 6   Therapeutic Communication

Chapter 7   Cultural and Ethnic Considerations

Chapter 8   Legal and Ethical Considerations

CHAPTER 1

History of Psychiatric Nursing

This chapter presents the history of psychiatric nursing, with an emphasis on nurses and organizations that have contributed to the development of psychiatric–mental health nursing. This background provides a basis for understanding the present status of psychiatric nursing.

Reading Assignment

Prior to beginning this assignment, please read Chapter 1, "History of Psychiatric Nursing."

Activities

Fill in the gaps with the correct information from Table 1–1 (pp. 8–10).

The Evolution of Psychiatric Nursing

Dates and Events	Type of Mental Health Treatment	Role of Psychiatric Nurse	Historical Figures	Significant Contributions
1773—First psychiatric hospital in America	Custodial care	Nonexistent		
1882—First training school for nurses in the United States	Custodial care	Attempts to create a safe environment		
1920s–1940s NIMH offered "integration grants"			First psychiatric nursing textbook	
1950–1960 Integration of psychiatric nursing into the curriculum				
1970s–1980s Decrease in federal funding			Major nursing leaders instructed in defining nursing practice within a changing health care system	
1990s–2000s Continued advances in technology				ANA revised standards of psychiatric–mental health nursing

The Evolution of Psychiatric Nursing (continued)

Dates and Events	Type of Mental Health Treatment	Role of Psychiatric Nurse	Historical Figures	Significant Contributions
2007–Future	Increased psychotropic use in children and adolescents; issues concerning suicide risk secondary to novel antidepressant use emerged and trends toward prescribing antidepressants declined as a result	Focus on violence, substance use disorders	Demographic changes associated with growing minority populations, particularly Hispanics and need to address cultural needs, improve communication, and decrease health disparities among diverse populations	Juvenile detention centers spend more than $420 million "warehousing" youth instead of providing mental health services

Using the content in the text, answer the following questions as clearly as you can and in your own words. Give examples to help clarify the information in your answer.

1. Describe the care of the mentally ill during the nineteenth century. What was the rationale for the care during this time? (pp. 7 and 11)

_____

_____

_____

_____

_____

2. The twentieth century is referred to as the "Era of Psychiatry." What do you think accounted for this? (p. 11)

_____

_____

_____

_____

_____

3. Compare the contributions of Sigmund Freud with those of Carl Jung. How do you see their concepts being used currently? (pp. 11–12)

_____

_____

_____

_____

_____

4. Delineate the four phases of the nurse-client relationship according to Hildegard Peplau. (p. 12)

_____

_____

_____

_____

_____

5. Explain the factors that led up to the passage of the national Mental Health Act of 1946. (p. 12)

_____

_____

_____

_____

_____

6. Define the "Decade of the Brain." How has psychiatric–mental nursing changed as a result? (p. 15)

_____

_____

_____

_____

_____

Critical Thinking Exercise

What do you see as the future of psychiatric–mental health nursing?

_____

_____

_____

_____

_____

Case Study

Suggested answers for Case Studies are provided in the Answers section at the back of this Study Guide.

Scenario:
After your History of Psychiatric Nursing class discussion, your classmate says to you, "I don't see why we have to study all this history of psychiatric nursing. We don't need to know this to take care of today's clients."

1. Your informed response should include what concept to support the need to study the history of psychiatric nursing?

_____

_____

_____

_____

2. Provide some examples from the eighteenth, nineteenth, and twentieth centuries to support your statement.

_____

_____

_____

_____

Self-Assessment Questions

Answers and rationales for Self-Assessment Questions are provided in the Answers section at the back of this Study Guide.

1. Nursing care of the 1920s–1940s was consistent with:
   a. The medical model
   b. Custodial care
   c. Therapeutic relationships
   d. Neuroscience

2. The purpose of nursing organizations for the advancement of psychiatric nursing includes:
   a. Protecting the profession
   b. Establishing standards of care
   c. Instituting licensure regulations
   d. Developing treatment options

3. Which comment by a nursing student in a psychiatric rotation would indicate that further teaching is needed?
   a. "I understand I need to establish a therapeutic relationship and environment."
   b. "I will be teaching positive coping skills."
   c. "I will be doing physical assessments."
   d. "I will be providing advice on various subjects."

4. When comparing commonly accepted treatments for psychiatric conditions in the eighteenth century with those popular in the Middle Ages, which of the following interventions is more applicable to the Middle Ages?
   a. Imprisonment
   b. Moral treatment
   c. Humane treatment
   d. Mesmerism

5. When comparing commonly held beliefs about the cause of mental illness in the early twentieth century with current theories of the cause of mental illness, early-twentieth-century theory included:
   a. Psychosexual concepts
   b. Neurobiology research
   c. Neurotransmitter abnormalities
   d. Brain disease

6. Which historical period initiated the first hospital that focused on the care of the mentally ill?
   a. The nineteenth century
   b. The Middle Ages
   c. The eighteenth century
   d. The twentieth century

7. In which historical period was the initiation of the therapeutic relationship emphasized?
    a. 1700s
    b. 1800s
    c. 1920–1940
    d. 1950s–1960s

8. Which best describes the deinstitutionalization movement?
    a. Use of the *Diagnostic and Statistical Manual of Mental Disorders* to standardize classification of mental illness
    b. Use of biological therapies to provide physical-based treatments for the mentally ill
    c. Release of chronically ill clients from institutions back into the community
    d. Promotion of mental health through federal provisions

9. A client is admitted with a history of using a variety of complementary therapies, such as acupuncture and St. John's wort for depression. The nurse:
    a. Must be familiar with the advantages and potential risks of complementary therapy
    b. Should teach the client that complementary therapies contradict conventional therapy
    c. Should support discharge if the client insists on continuing the use of St. John's wort
    d. Should deny access to the client's acupuncturist

—NOTES—

CHAPTER 2

Concepts of Psychiatric Care: Therapeutic Models

This chapter presents concepts that are utilized in psychiatric–mental health nursing. As a result of this exposure, you should be able to relate to the role that theories play in understanding their relationship to psychiatric–mental health nursing.

Reading Assignment

Prior to beginning this assignment, please read Chapter 2, "Concepts of Psychiatric Care: Therapeutic Models."

Activities

Using the content in the text, answer the following questions as clearly as you can and in your own words. Give examples to help clarify the information in your answer.

1. Explain the difference between *eros* and *thanatos* in terms of their significance. (pp. 31–32, 34)

    _____

    _____

    _____

    _____

    _____

2. Define primary thinking. Give examples. (p. 34)

    _____

    _____

    _____

    _____

    _____

3. Differentiate among the id, ego, and superego. (p. 34)

_____

_____

_____

_____

_____

4. Differentiate between primary process thinking and secondary process thinking. (p. 34)

_____

_____

_____

_____

_____

5. What are the purposes of defense mechanisms? (pp. 34–36)

_____

_____

_____

_____

_____

6. How can one apply interpersonal, psychoanalytical, and behavioral theories to nursing practice? (pp. 38, 41, 46)

_____

_____

_____

_____

_____

7. Explain Harry Stack Sullivan's theory of interpersonal relationships. (p. 41)

_____

_____

_____

_____

_____

8. Identify the stages of cognitive development according to Piaget. (pp. 49–50)

_____

_____

_____

_____

_____

9. Relate Piaget's stages of development to the nursing process. (p. 50)

_____

_____

_____

_____

_____

10. List the phases of Sullivan's theory. Describe the level of interacting in each of these. (Table 2–5, p. 41)

_____

_____

_____

_____

_____

11. Describe three interventions to challenge distortions in clients who are anxious or depressed. (pp. 46–48)

_____

_____

_____

_____

_____

12. Fill in the correct information to identify how the listed models may be applied to nursing.

Model	Basic Concepts	Application to Nursing
Systems theory (pp. 59–60)		
Human needs theory (pp. 60–61)		
Wellness-illness continuum (pp. 61–63)		
Stress adaptation models (pp. 63–64)		

13. Explain the following nursing models. How can they be applied to psychiatric–mental health nursing?

a. Neuman's systems model (p. 64)

_____

_____

1. Person_____

_____

2. Nursing_____

_____

3. Health_____

_____

4. Environment_____

_____

b. Orem's self-care model (p. 65)

_____

_____

1. Person _____

_____

2. Nursing _____

_____

3. Health _____

_____

4. Environment _____

_____

c. Orlando's needs-oriented theory (p. 65)

_____

_____

1. Person _____

_____

2. Nursing _____

_____

3. Health _____

_____

4. Environment _____

_____

d. Roy's model of adaptation (p. 65)

_____

_____

1. Person _____

_____

2. Nursing _____

_____

3. Health _____

_____

4. Environment _____

_____

e. Peplau's interpersonal theory (p. 66)

_____

_____

1. Person _____

_____

2. Nursing_____

_____

3. Health_____

_____

4. Environment_____

_____

Case Study

Suggested answers for Case Studies are provided in the Answers section at the back of this Study Guide.

Scenario:
In the morning report on the adolescent unit, a client is described as out of control and nonadherent with the treatment plan. One of the professional staff members states, "The behavior of the client is a product of where he came from."

1. To which theoretical model is the staff member referring?

_____

_____

_____

_____

_____

2. How would use of this model help determine a plan of care for the client?

_____

_____

_____

_____

_____

Self-Assessment Questions

Answers and rationales for Self-Assessment Questions are provided in the Answers section at the back of this Study Guide.

1. An elderly client has refused to bathe for over a week. She has worn the same food-stained clothing for several days. Using a cognitive model in assisting her to shower and change into fresh clothing, what approach would be used?

    a.   Provide limited options for her to choose from, such as when to shower and what to wear

    b.   Negotiate a solution

    c.   Teach the importance and benefits of regular hygiene practices

    d.   Use medication to sedate the client

2. The primary pharmacologic target in schizophrenia is which important neurotransmitter?

    a.   Serotonin

    b.   Gamma aminobutyric acid (GABA)

    c.   Dopamine

    d.   Norepinephrine

3. A nurse who primarily employs Peplau's interpersonal theory:
   a. Provides a safe milieu
   b. Facilitates the therapeutic effects of the nurse-client relationship
   c. Focuses on the role of neurotransmitters in mental illness
   d. Analyzes client behavior using defense mechanisms

4. While working with a family of a young out-of-control child, the nurse teaches the parents to use positive reinforcement with tokens. This approach is typical of which theoretical perspective?
   a. Psychoanalytical
   b. Neurobiological
   c. Interpersonal social
   d. Behavioral

5. A person who states, "I know where I am going in life. I have a plan to go to college and get a degree in engineering. I enjoy working with my hands and believe I can be a contributing member of society," is indicating successful fulfillment of which of Erikson's eight stages of ego development?
   a. Initiative–guilt
   b. Trust–mistrust
   c. Autonomy–doubt, shame
   d. Intimacy–role confusion

6. Which of the following statements is consistent with the superego?
   a. "I shouldn't buy this expensive dress."
   b. "This is the perfect dress for my new job interview. It doesn't matter what it costs."
   c. "I don't deserve to buy this dress until I prove I can get a job."
   d. "Credit cards are made just for this reason: to get what I want when I want it."

7. A client explains that he is not responsible for being fired because his supervisor is ineffective. This is an example of which defense mechanism?
   a. Denial
   b. Repression
   c. Intellectualization
   d. Displacement

8. A person who earns more than the national average salary, saves all his money, buys all his clothes at thrift stores, and shops for the very cheapest grocery brands may be fixated on which of Freud's stages of psychosexual growth and development?
   a. Oral
   b. Anal
   c. Phallic
   d. Latency

9. An infant is observed giggling and clinging lovingly to her mother. This assessment correlates with which therapeutic model?

    a.   Neurobiological

    b.   Interpersonal social

    c.   Psychoanalytical

    d.   Cognitive

10. A parent uses a "time out" technique for disciplining his children. This is an example of which operant conditioning concept?

    a.   Positive reinforcement

    b.   Negative reinforcement

    c.   Punishment

    d.   Classic conditioning

—NOTES—

CHAPTER 3

Interfacing Biological-Behavioral Concepts into Psychiatric Nursing Practice

This chapter presents the major neurobiological and behavioral models. The student is also introduced to the interrelatedness of human behavior and brain function.

Reading Assignment

Prior to beginning this assignment, please read Chapter 3, "Interfacing Biological-Behavioral Concepts into Psychiatric Nursing Practice."

Activities

Using the content in the text, answer the following questions as clearly as you can and in your own words. Give examples to help clarify the information in your answer.

1. Explain the functions of the central nervous system. (p. 79)

_____

_____

_____

_____

_____

2. State the differences between the neurodegenerative processes and the neurochemical processes. (pp. 79–81)

_____

_____

_____

_____

_____

3. Give four examples of excitatory neurotransmitters. (p. 81)

_____

_____

_____

_____

_____

4. Give one example of inhibitory neurotransmitters. (p. 81)

_____

_____

_____

_____

_____

5. Define humoral immunity. (p. 81)

_____

_____

_____

_____

_____

6. Explain the difference among twin, adoption, and family studies, as well as their relevance in the understanding of genetics. (p. 82)

_____

_____

_____

_____

_____

7. Give four examples of environmental factors that are believed to buffer or protect genetically vulnerable clients. (p. 82)

_____

_____

_____

_____

_____

8. List the major treatment modalities that are used in the integration of the biological and behavioral aspects of mental illness. (pp. 83–84)

_____

_____

_____

_____

_____

Case Study

Suggested answers for Case Studies are provided in the Answers section at the back of this Study Guide.

Scenario:
During an interdisciplinary care conference for a client with an acute and severe psychiatric disorder, the primary nurse states, "The client's father and paternal grandmother also have severe mental illness. It appears our client may have a genetic basis for his diagnosis."

1. To which theoretical model would the primary nurse be referring?

   _____

   _____

   _____

2. What support courses in your curriculum support the understanding of this theoretical model?

   _____

   _____

   _____

3. What approaches may the interdisciplinary team consider in planning care for a client with a genetic basis for his illness?

   _____

   _____

   _____

Self-Assessment Questions

Answers and rationales for Self-Assessment Questions are provided in the Answers section at the back of this Study Guide.

1. A client with severe anxiety is being assessed in the community mental health center. The nurse understands that which of the following neurotransmitter abnormalities is implicated in anxiety disorders?
   a. Increased dopamine
   b. Decreased norepinephrine
   c. Decreased GABA
   d. Decreased acetylcholine

2. A client with depression is suicidal. He has no appetite and has difficulty sleeping. The most appropriate explanation for his illness involves which of the following?
   a. Dysregulation of a neurotransmitter such as serotonin
   b. Hormone abnormalities of the pituitary gland
   c. Decreased GABA
   d. Excess impulses of the afferent neurons

3. A client asks the nurse why the psychiatrist ordered an electroencephalography (EEG) test. The teaching should include which of the following?

    a. The EEG test is used to identify anomalies in brain rhythm such as in epilepsy, neoplasm, stroke, or metabolic or degenerative diseases.

    b. The EEG test can determine possible lesions in the brain.

    c. The EEG test measures glucose metabolism, oxygen use, blood flow, and neurotransmitter interaction in the brain.

    d. The EEG test can detect brain edema, ischemia, infection, or trauma in the brain.

4. What statement by a depressed client would indicate that teaching is successful?

    a. "My brain probably does not have enough serotonin."

    b. "I have excess dopamine in parts of my brain."

    c. "My parents likely used double-bind communication when I was younger."

    d. "I have a hypothalamic dysfunction."

5. A family asks the nurse to help them understand their mother's recent Alzheimer's diagnosis. The nurse should include in the teaching plan which of the following?

    a. The mother's limbic system is overstimulated.

    b. The ventricles of the brain have shrunk as a result of normal aging.

    c. The mother has experienced some form of major brain trauma.

    d. Alzheimer's is a neurodegenerative disorder.

6. A student is having difficulty understanding the purpose of twin studies associated with research on mental illness. Another student asks, "How is this going to help us understand how to take care of clients?" What is the best response to the classmate's question?

    a. Twin studies help determine the frequency of psychiatric disorders.

    b. Twin studies indicate that if one person in a family develops a disorder, then the other will too.

    c. Twin studies makes it easier to find subjects with similar disorders.

    d. Twin studies can help determine whether genetics or environment influences the precipitating factors of mental illnesses.

7. Which of the following questions by a nurse indicates that the nurse is using more than a neurobiological approach to care?

    a. "Is there a history of mental illness in the family?"

    b. "What medications are you currently taking?"

    c. "What are the stressors in your life?"

    d. "How frequently do you experience these headaches?"

CHAPTER 4

Foundations of Psychiatric Nursing

This chapter shows the relationship between stress and adaptation and the role of the psychiatric nurse in prevention of mental illness.

Reading Assignment

Prior to beginning this assignment, please read Chapter 4, "Foundations of Psychiatric Nursing."

Activities

Using the content in the text, answer the following questions as clearly as you can and in your own words. Give examples to help clarify the information in your answer.

1. List the three stages of prevention in mental health nursing. Explain the role of the nurse during each stage. (pp. 99–100)

   _____

   _____

   _____

   _____

   _____

2. What are the three phases of the general adaptation syndrome? Identify the body's response during each phase. (p. 102)

   Phase   **Body's Response**

   1. _____   _____

   2. _____   _____

   3. _____   _____

3. List the various psychological defense mechanisms, define them, and give examples. (p. 103)

Defense Mechanism	Definition	Example

4. Explain the criteria that are relevant for each axis of the DSM organizational framework. (p. 106)

Axis	Explanation
_____	_____
_____	_____
_____	_____
_____	_____
_____	_____

Case Study

Suggested answers for Case Studies are provided in the Answers section at the back of this Study Guide.

Scenario:
The admitting nurse gives a report on a new client and states, "She is a 27-year-old female with depression, and she is suicidal. She has been a diabetic since age 14. Her family describes her as having always been a quiet, withdrawn person, and she has no friends. She socializes with family members only. She lived alone and has had only minimum-wage jobs. Recently she was fired from her last job and was evicted from her apartment for failure to pay rent. She is currently living with her parents, who state that she lies in bed all day, rarely bathes, refuses meals, and speaks only when spoken to."

1. Which data correspond with Axis I of the *DSM-IV-TR*?

   _____

   _____

2. Which data correspond with Axis II of the *DSM-IV-TR*?

   _____

   _____

3. What cluster will be considered in the Axis II diagnosis?

_____

_____

_____

4. Which data correspond with Axis III of the *DSM-IV-TR*?

_____

_____

_____

5. Which data correspond with Axis IV of the *DSM-IV-TR*?

_____

_____

_____

6. Which data correspond with Axis V of the *DSM-IV-TR*?

_____

_____

_____

7. What defense mechanisms might the client be using?

_____

_____

_____

Self-Assessment Questions

Answers and rationales for Self-Assessment Questions are provided in the Answers section at the back of this Study Guide.

1. A psychiatric nurse meets with the clients in the community health center. She approaches a new client and states, "I am the nurse who will be working with you. I look forward to working with you." These comments are most closely associated with which of the essential qualities of psychiatric nurses?
   a. Therapeutic use of self
   b. Empathy
   c. Self-awareness
   d. Maturity

2. An advanced-practice psychiatric registered nurse has identified the educational need of the client. Which of Krupnick's four phases of the consultation-liaison process has the nurse accomplished?
   a. Entry
   b. Diagnosis
   c. Response/intervention
   d. Closure and evaluation

3. A community mental health client voices her concerns regarding a news item on CNN. She states, "Those poor people who have lost their homes. I just cannot get that image out of my mind." Which of the following best describes the individual's assessment of this situation?

   a. Primary appraisal-stress-injurious

   b. Primary appraisal-stress-challenging

   c. Primary appraisal-irrelevant-challenging

   d. Secondary appraisal-stress-hazardous

4. A client in outpatient therapy has been working on becoming more independent following a divorce. Over the course of therapy, the client has said the following: "I can see things are getting better now. I know my trigger points and can see when I need a little help. Before I make a decision now, I make a list of options before deciding what to do." Which of the coping behaviors from the Jalowiec Coping Scales are associated with the client's comments? Select all that apply.

   a. Get mad

   b. Handle problem in steps

   c. Discuss the problem

   d. Withdraw from the situation

   e. Try anything

   f. Hope for improvement

   g. Maintain control

   h. Make use of past experiences

5. After a session with his psychiatrist in which the client's behavior was confronted, the client is seen yelling at the new receptionist about leaving the newspaper unfolded. Which major defense mechanism is the client displaying?

   a. Displacement

   b. Denial

   c. Rationalization

   d. Intellectualization

6. A client has recently lost a child due to a terminal illness. Which statement by the nurse would indicate empathy?

   a. "I know you are feeling very depressed right now. I know anyone who has lost someone close can get depressed."

   b. "I feel very sorry for you. No one should have to lose a loved one."

   c. "I can understand that you are feeling very sad right now. I imagine it is a very difficult time for you."

   d. "You need to take some time off to process this."

7. A nurse is conscious of his own nonverbal behaviors while communicating with the client. When the conversation is sad, the nurse has a sober expression on his face. When the conversation is lighthearted, the nurse has a smile. In this congruence between verbal and nonverbal communication, the nurse is conveying:

   a. Warmth

   b. Genuineness

   c. Sympathy

   d. Rapport

8. A client continues to consume alcohol on a daily basis even though the client has numerous physical and social problems related to drinking. This is an example of which defense mechanism?

   a. Displacement

   b. Denial

   c. Intellectualization

   d. Projection

9. A nursing student tells her classmates, "I don't have to study for the next psychiatric nursing test. That content was all covered in my introduction to psychology course." This is an example of which defense mechanism?

   a. Displacement

   b. Introjection

   c. Rationalization

   d. Repression

10. A client's history reads: 35-year-old male with depression, mental retardation, diabetes mellitus, mild psychosocial stressors, and limited functioning. Which axis of the *DSM-IV-TR* is associated with the mental retardation data?

   a. Axis I

   b. Axis II

   c. Axis III

   d. Axis IV

—NOTES—

CHAPTER 5

The Nursing Process

This chapter presents the nursing process as it relates to psychiatric nursing standards. The role of the nurse is highlighted as each stage of the process is identified.

Reading Assignment

Prior to beginning this assignment, please read Chapter 5, "The Nursing Process."

Activities

Using the content in the text, answer the following questions as clearly as you can and, if possible, in your own words. Give examples, as indicated, to help clarify the information in your answer.

1. List the major benefits of a spiritual assessment. (pp. 139–140)

    _____

    _____

    _____

    _____

    _____

Case Study

Suggested answers for Case Studies are provided in the Answers section at the back of this Study Guide.

Scenario:
A client is admitted with complaints of feeling depressed.

1. What are typical symptoms that might be expected of a client who complains of depression?

    _____

    _____

_____

_____

_____

2. List several questions that the nurse should ask in the assessment of a client complaining of depression.

_____

_____

_____

_____

_____

3. What nursing diagnoses are often associated with depressed clients?

_____

_____

_____

_____

_____

Self-Assessment Questions

Answers and rationales for Self-Assessment Questions are provided in the Answers section at the back of this Study Guide.

1. During assessment, a nurse asks the client to state what she ate for breakfast. This question assesses which of the client's higher brain functions?

   a. Memory

   b. Cognition

   c. Visuospatial ability

   d. Intellectual ability

2. A nursing student laughs when she hears the nurse ask a client the meaning of the phrase "A bird in the hand is worth two in the bush." The student should know that the purpose of such a question is to:

   a. Determine a client's ability to concentrate

   b. Estimate a client's intelligence

   c. Test for the ability to perform abstract reasoning

   d. Examine the client's ability to store and retrieve information

3. A client asks the nurse why the medical technician drew blood for a thyroid test. The nurse's response should include which of the following?

   a. Some disorders of the thyroid can be similar to symptoms associated with psychiatric disorders.

   b. The thyroid helps regulate neurotransmitters.

   c. Before giving any psychotropic medication, the psychiatrist needs to know if the thyroid can metabolize the medication.

   d. The thyroid test can help determine if there will be any side effects from any medication.

4. Which of the following comments would be essential in collecting data regarding the spiritual assessment?

    a. "What religion do you follow?"

    b. "Describe for me the meaning and significance of spiritual or religious practices to you."

    c. "When do you usually attend church services?"

    d. "What religious holidays do you celebrate?"

5. A depressed client has slept through the night for 8 hours and has gained 10 of the 30 pounds that he lost. This information is associated with which stage of the nursing process?

    a. Assessment

    b. Nursing diagnosis

    c. Implementation

    d. Evaluation

6. A client states, "I am always in trouble. I am either in debt or breaking up with my boyfriend." Which of the following nursing diagnoses is most appropriate for this client?

    a. Self-esteem, low

    b. Ineffective coping

    c. Social isolation

    d. Impaired social interaction

7. Assuming that a client has all of the following nursing diagnoses, which one has the highest priority?

    a. Sleep pattern, disturbed

    b. Spiritual distress

    c. Violence, risk for self-directed

    d. Disturbed body image

8. What is an appropriate nursing diagnosis related to a client who hears voices that no one else can hear?

    a. Disturbed sensory perception

    b. Disturbed body image

    c. Disturbed thought processes

    d. Disturbed personal identity

—NOTES—

CHAPTER 6

Therapeutic Communication

In this chapter, the causative factors affecting communication patterns (which include neurobiological, genetic, psychosocial, and developmental issues) are addressed, as well as types of communication, communication theories, and the factors that contribute to patterns of communication. The chapter also addresses some therapeutic communication techniques and the phases of the nurse-client relationship.

Reading Assignment

Prior to beginning this assignment, please read Chapter 6, "Therapeutic Communication."

Activities

Using the content in the text, answer the following questions as clearly as you can and in your own words. Give examples to help clarify the information in your answer.

1. Explain the difference between encoding and decoding. Give examples of each. (p. 154)

    _____

    _____

    _____

    _____

    _____

2. Fill in the correct information from Table 6–1. (p. 153)

Communication with Clients across the Life Span

	Developmental Influences	Age-Specific Behaviors	Age-Specific Communication
Prenatal	Genetics, _____, _____ Damage during birth process		
Infancy	Mental retardation, _____- _____, _____, sensory deprivation (aloof care givers), _____		

Communication with Clients across the Life Span (continued)

	Developmental Influences	**Age-Specific Behaviors**	**Age-Specific Communication**
Childhood	Autism, _____, sensory deprivation	Limited vocabulary that _____ _____ _____, tense	_____ _____ accepting approach
Adolescence	Psychosis _____ _____ _____	_____ _____ _____	_____ _____ _____
Adulthood	_____ _____ _____	Cognitive function _____	Establish rapport, _____ _____
Late adulthood	Medical conditions, _____ _____	_____ _____	_____ _____

3. List examples of each aspect of nonverbal behavior in the nurse, in terms of body language, that convey warmth, caring, and calmness to clients. (pp. 155–156.)

    a. _____

    b. _____

    c. _____

    d. _____

    e. _____

    f. _____

4. List the four phases of the nurse-client relationship according to Peplau. Describe some elements of each phase. (pp. 166–170)

    Phase   **Description**

    1. _____   _____

                                                _____

                                                _____

    2. _____   _____

                                                _____

                                                _____

                                                _____

    3. _____   _____

                                                _____

                                                _____

                                                _____

    4. _____   _____

                                                _____

                                                _____

Case Study

Suggested answers for Case Studies are provided in the Answers section at the back of this Study Guide.

Scenario:
A new psychiatric assistant is in orientation on your unit. As the RN on the unit, you observe the following inter-action: The psychiatric assistant stands over the sitting client, who is paranoid. The two are in an alcove area of the unit in which there is only one exit. The staff member is standing in this exit. The client is heard to say, "They are out to get me. I am sure that they will find me in here. I am not safe anywhere." The staff member is heard to say, "Tell me who they are and I will watch out for them."

1. Identify nonverbal behavior by the staff member that is nontherapeutic.

   _____

   _____

   _____

   _____

   _____

2. Analyze the staff member's verbal comment. Identify whether it is therapeutic or nontherapeutic.

   _____

   _____

   _____

   _____

   _____

3. What nursing diagnoses are oftentimes associated with a paranoid client such as this?

   _____

   _____

   _____

   _____

   _____

4. What would be a therapeutic response in this situation?

   _____

   _____

   _____

   _____

   _____

Self-Assessment Questions

Answers and rationales for Self-Assessment Questions are provided in the Answers section at the back of this Study Guide.

1. A nurse interviews a new admission at the nurse's station, keeps her notebook between the nurse and the client, and often asks the client to repeat information. An appropriate assessment of the nurse's nonverbal communication is that the nurse:

   a. Wants to record all information correctly

   b. Is concerned about her appearance and professional image

   c. Would prefer to be someplace else

   d. Considers social interactions important

2. A nurse's interview with a client has reached a sensitive subject; however, it is time for the nurse to lead a regularly scheduled anger management group. What action is most appropriate for the nurse?

   a. Cancel the anger management group

   b. Help the client to connect with another qualified individual

   c. Apologize to the client and start the group as scheduled

   d. Bring the client conversation to closure

3. Which of the following statements by the nurse indicates therapeutic reflection?

   a. "You look angry. Let's talk about that."

   b. "I'd like to know more about what brought you to the hospital."

   c. "So you are saying it wasn't your fault?"

   d. "How are you doing today?"

4. Which of the following statements by the nurse is most therapeutic for a client who is seeing things that no one else sees?

   a. "It is Sue. I am your nurse today."

   b. "I do not see any animals in your room, but there are some clothes lying on the floor."

   c. "What exactly are you seeing?"

   d. "How are you feeling?"

5. A hospitalized client states, "Will they find me in here? I don't feel safe anywhere." Which of the following responses by the nurse is therapeutic?

   a. "Perhaps you should consider how that sounds to others."

   b. "I find it hard to believe you have others after you."

   c. "What makes you say that?"

   d. "Of course it is safe in here."

6. The client says, "Whenever I ask the nurses for something, they ignore me." In response, the nurse says, "I think we know best for the clients here." This nontherapeutic response is an example of:

   a. Giving recognition

   b. Focusing

   c. Verbalizing the implied

   d. Rejecting

7. During couples' counseling, a husband occasionally becomes unreasonably angry. Which of the following comments by the nurse therapist would be therapeutic?

   a. "You were very inappropriate in expressing your anger."

   b. "You were quite angry just now, raising your voice, pounding on the table, and demanding an answer."

   c. "Showing your anger that way is counterproductive."

   d. "I don't see any progress when you have these outbursts."

8. The following exchange between nurse and client takes place.

   Nurse: From what you have said, I am wondering if one of the areas for you to work on is an issue with low self-esteem.

   Client: I don't know about self-esteem, but if you mean I don't feel very good about myself right now, then yes.

   This exchange is indicative of which phase of the nurse-client relationship?

   a. Orientation phase

   b. Identification phase

   c. Exploitation phase

   d. Resolution phase

9. Which of the following nurse statements indicates self-awareness?

   a. "The client looks just like my older brother."

   b. "I must act professional at all times during my interactions with clients."

   c. "The client is using projection at this time."

   d. "I think the client is actively hallucinating."

10. Which of the following statements indicates active listening?

   a. "It sounds as though you are angry about your daughter's choice of boyfriend."

   b. "It is normal for your daughter to want to make some of her own choices."

   c. "It might help to think back when you were a teenager and remember what that was like for you."

   d. "Tell me more about how your daughter defied your request not to see her boyfriend."

—NOTES—

CHAPTER 7

Cultural and Ethnic Considerations

This chapter gives worldview perspectives of different cultural groups. Components of a cultural assessment are also addressed, as well as ethnopsychopharmacology.

Reading Assignment

Prior to beginning this assignment, please read Chapter 7, "Cultural and Ethnic Considerations."

Case Study

Suggested answers for Case Studies are provided in the Answers section at the back of this Study Guide.

Scenario:
A recent immigrant from a South American country is admitted to the unit with a diagnosis of schizopnia. Although she speaks English, she uses a language of guttural sounds that her family does not recognize. She admits to seeing things that no one else sees and hearing things no one else hears. She is seen muttering to herself and using nonverbal forms of communication toward no one in particular. The family is very concerned and asks questions about how to approach her.

1. What culturally competent concepts should be included in the family teaching?

   _____

   _____

   _____

   _____

   _____

2. What questions by the nurse would help assess this client in a culturally competent manner?

   _____

   _____

_____

_____

_____

3. What activity by the nurse is essential when interacting with clients from cultures other than the nurse's own?

_____

_____

_____

_____

_____

Self-Assessment Questions

Answers and rationales for Self-Assessment Questions are provided in the Answers section at the back of this Study Guide.

1. A client with a culturally diverse background is being admitted by the nurse. It is essential that the nurse understand that:

   a. Most individuals want the same things under similar circumstances.

   b. Culture does not affect the manifestation of psychiatric symptoms.

   c. A nurse's worldview influences the therapeutic relationship.

   d. The nurse should use projection to better understand the client's behavior.

2. A client who is most concerned about her "things" being locked away and out of her possession would most likely be associated with which of Nichols' worldview perspectives?

   a. European American cultural groups

   b. Latino/Hispanic American cultural groups

   c. Asian American cultural groups

   d. Native American cultural groups

3. A client of a culturally diverse background responds unexpectedly to a common psychotropic medication. In teaching this client about the situation, it is important to include:

   a. Concepts related to ethnopsychopharmacology

   b. The importance of taking the medication as prescribed

   c. Consequences of not taking medication on time

   d. Side effects specific to the client's ethnic background

4. A client of African American culture has developed a severe mental illness. The nurse understands that:

   a. The incidence of mental illness in African Americans is similar to the incidence in European Americans.

   b. Internal differences account for any difference in incidence between European Americans and African Americans.

c.   "Keeping face" within the African American community contributes to a lower incidence of mental illness.

d.   The incidence of mental illness in African Americans is higher due to socioeconomic differences.

5.   A European American and an Asian American are both given identical doses of an anxiolytic medication. Even though the two clients are similar in height and weight, the Asian American client develops symptoms of toxicity. To what is this response attributed?

a.   The Asian American took more than the prescribed amount of drug.

b.   The Asian American is dehydrated.

c.   The European American skipped a dose of medication.

d.   The Asian American metabolized the medication at a slower rate.

—NOTES—

CHAPTER 8

Legal and Ethical Considerations

Legal and ethical aspects of psychiatric care are presented in this chapter. Historical events that have affected the course of psychiatric–mental health nursing are introduced. This chapter also includes criteria for admission to a psychiatric facility as well as the nurse's role in the prevention of litigation for malpractice issues.

Reading Assignment

Prior to beginning this assignment, please read Chapter 8, "Legal and Ethical Considerations."

Activities

Using the content in the text, answer the following questions as clearly as you can and in your own words. Give examples, if appropriate, to help clarify the information in your answer.

1. Explain the nurse's role in the following. (pp. 205–206)

   a. Transfer _____

   _____

   _____

   _____

   b. Elopement _____

   _____

   _____

   _____

   c. Discharge _____

   _____

   _____

   _____

2. List the characteristics that may be evident in an individual who is being assessed for serious intent to harm others. (Figure 8–6, p. 207)

a. _____

b. _____

c. _____

d. _____

e. _____

f. _____

g. _____

Case Study

Suggested answers for Case Studies are provided in the Answers section at the back of this Study Guide.

Scenario:
An individual arrives at the emergency department of a large hospital saying he is schizophrenic. He denies hallucinations, appears well fed, and has clean clothes. His speech is rambling and he laughs inappropriately.

1. Does he meet the criteria for involuntary admission?

_____

_____

_____

_____

_____

2. Why or why not?

_____

_____

_____

_____

_____

3. Must the hospital admit him?

_____

_____

_____

_____

_____

4. Why or why not?

_____

_____

_____

5. Should the hospital admit him? Base your answer on an ethical concept.

_____

_____

_____

_____

_____

Self-Assessment Questions

Answers and rationales for Self-Assessment Questions are provided in the Answers section at the back of this Study Guide.

1. A client is placed in the quiet room against his will and without following hospital procedure. The nurse responsible for this action may be found guilty of:
    a. Assault
    b. Battery
    c. Slander
    d. Negligence

2. A client is coerced into taking his medication against his wishes. The nurse does this by stating, "You have to take this medication. If you don't, the doctor will discharge you." Which element of legal consent is being violated in this situation?
    a. The client must be capable of consenting.
    b. The client must have the ability to refuse consent.
    c. The client must have adequate information.
    d. The consent must not be illegal.

3. The client asks the medication nurse to explain the purpose of one of the medications. The nurse responds, "Your doctor wants you to have this medication to get better." This response violates which ethical principle?
    a. The client has the right to informed consent.
    b. The client has the right to refuse treatment.
    c. The nurse has violated the principle of justice.
    d. The nurse has violated the principle of beneficence.

4. A client is a serious danger to himself and others, and he has a severe mental illness. Because the client refuses treatment, a hearing must be conducted. The rationale for the hearing is:
    a. The client has a right to due process.
    b. The client has disability rights.
    c. The client has a right to treatment.
    d. The client has a right to informed consent.

5. A client with a mental illness that is in remission is denied employment based on having a mental illness. This situation violates which client right?

    a. The client has a right to due process.

    b. The client has disability rights.

    c. The client has a right to treatment.

    d. The client has a right to informed consent.

6. A state-supported outpatient clinic denies admission to a client with a mental disorder because it does not offer mental health services. The clinic is:

    a. Open to a lawsuit because it must provide all services

    b. Not open to a lawsuit because it cannot be forced to create treatment where none exists

    c. Open to a lawsuit because it violates disability rights

    d. Not open to a lawsuit because the client should seek services at an inpatient facility

7. The person on the phone asks to speak to a particular client. The caller states, "He is my husband." The nurse's most appropriate response is:

    a. "I will get your husband to the phone."

    b. "I will give you his direct phone number."

    c. "Please call him back this afternoon."

    d. "I can neither confirm nor deny that the person you wish to speak to is here."

8. A new medication with which the nurse is unfamiliar has been ordered for a client. The medication nurse should:

    a. Give the medication as prescribed

    b. Hold the medication until the nurse has looked up the drug

    c. Call to see if the medication can be changed

    d. Ask the pharmacist which side effects to watch for after administration

9. A client who has shown marked improvement in his mental illness is no longer considered a danger to himself or others. His admission status has been changed from involuntary to voluntary. This means that he can now do which of the following that he could not do while under involuntary status?

    a. Call his attorney

    b. Receive phone calls

    c. Refuse treatment, including medications

    d. Wear his own clothing

10. In which of the following situations is the nurse breaching confidentiality?

    a. The nurse in the emergency department calls the mother of a college student to inform her that the student has made a suicide attempt.

    b. The nurse informs a parent that an adult child has threatened to hurt the parent.

    c. The nurse reports a suspected abuse of an elderly parent by an adult son.

    d. The nurse discusses a client's symptoms with a co-worker in another area of the hospital.

UNIT 2

Response to Stressors across the Life Span

Chapter 9   The Client with a Depressive Disorder

Chapter 10   The Client with a Bipolar Disorder

Chapter 11   The Client with an Anxiety Disorder

Chapter 12   The Client with a Somatization Disorder

Chapter 13   The Client with a Stress-Related Disorder

Chapter 14   The Client with Schizophrenia and Other Psychotic Disorders

Chapter 15   The Client with a Personality Disorder

Chapter 16   The Client with Delirium, Dementia, Amnestic, and Other Congnitive Disorders

Chapter 17   The Client with Attention-Deficit Disorder

Chapter 18   The Client with a Dissociative Disorder

Chapter 19   The Client at Risk of Suicidal and Self-Destructive Behaviors

Chapter 20   The Client Exhibiting Agression, Hostility, and Violence

Chapter 21   The Client with a Substance-Related Disorder

Chapter 22   The Client with an Eating Disorder

Chapter 23   The Client with a Sleep Disorder

Chapter 24   The Client with a Sexual Disorder

Chapter 25   The Client Who Survives Violence

CHAPTER 9

The Client with a Depressive Disorder

In this chapter, the student begins to address major psychiatric disorders and the way in which the *DSM-IV-TR* is used for purposes of classification. Various causative theories of depression are discussed, and signs and symptoms across the life span are presented.

Reading Assignment

Prior to beginning this assignment, please read Chapter 9, "The Client with a Depressive Disorder."

Activities

Using the content in the text, answer the following questions as clearly as you can and in your own words. Give examples, if appropriate, to help clarify the information in your answer.

1. Fill in the correct information from Table 9–7. (p. 243)

Differentiating Characteristics of Depression and Dementia

Clinical Features	Depression	Dementia
Onset		
Precursors		
Psychiatric history		
Cognitive impairment		
Orientation		
Memory		
Learning capacity		
Mental status results		
Sense of distress		
Affect		
Response to treatment		

2. Fill in the correct information from Table 9–8. (p. 245)

Manifestations of Normal Grief across the Life Span

Children	Adolescents	Adults	Older Adults

3. What are the risk factors for pathological grief reactions? Give examples of each. (Table 9–9, p. 246)

Risk Factor	**Example**
a. _____	_____
	_____
b. _____	_____
	_____
c. _____	_____
	_____
d. _____	_____
	_____

4. Name the four phases of pharmacologic treatment to manage depression, and indicate the interventions that occur during these phases. (pp. 247–248)

Phase	**Interventions**
a. _____	_____
	_____
b. _____	_____
	_____
c. _____	_____
	_____
d. _____	_____
	_____

Case Study

Suggested answers for Case Studies are provided in the Answers section at the back of this Study Guide.

Scenario:

An older client is brought in by family members for an assessment. He presents with the following complaints: He awakes most nights at 2 or 3 a.m. unable to fall back to sleep. He has lost his appetite and has lost at least 20 pounds in the last 3 months. He is uninterested in seeing his grandchildren, even though he used to love to attend all of their school events. He states, "It is no use. There is no reason to go on any longer. I should have invested more when I was younger so my kids would have something when I am gone. I don't really care about anything anymore." He appears disheveled, with his clothing dirty and hanging loosely. He is unshaven, with downcast eyes and a blank expression on his face.

1. What are the key symptoms that support the diagnosis of depression?

_____

_____

_____

_____

_____

2. What additional assessment questions must be asked?

_____

_____

_____

_____

_____

3. What is the priority nursing diagnosis?

_____

_____

_____

_____

_____

4. What other nursing diagnosis should be considered for this client?

_____

_____

_____

_____

_____

5. What treatment plan would you expect with this client?

_____

_____

_____

_____

_____

Self-Assessment Questions

Answers and rationales for Self-Assessment Questions are provided in the Answers section at the back of this Study Guide.

1. Which statement by a depressed client taking an antidepressant would indicate that further teaching is necessary?
   a. "Once I start taking medication, I should begin to feel better within a day or two."
   b. "My appetite should improve once my depression is resolved."
   c. "My medications work on the synaptic gap in my brain."
   d. "I can expect to be able to sleep through the night again once I begin to feel better."

2. A client is taking escitalopram (Lexapro) for depression. Which of the following should be reflected in your teaching to the client?
   a. It increases serotonin levels.
   b. It decreases norepinephrine levels.
   c. It increases dopamine levels.
   d. It increases cortisol levels.

3. A cause of a client's depression may be explained by reinforcement theory. Which of the following statements is consistent with reinforcement theory?
   a. The client learned depressive behaviors by seeing her mother exhibit them while the client was growing up.
   b. The client has experienced a significant loss in the unexpected death of her husband.
   c. The client has a faulty information processing defect.
   d. Depression is maintained through sympathy from others.

4. A depressed client states, "I should never have let my dog run out on the street. Now it's my fault that he is dead." Select the one best response by the nurse.
   a. "I understand that you feel bad about the accident."
   b. "You are not a failure for this one mistake."
   c. "What proof do you have that it is your fault?"
   d. "I'd like to hear you list those things that you are very good at doing."

5. In teaching a client alternative ways of looking at a situation, which of the following statements by the client would indicate that further teaching is necessary?

    a. "It is helpful for me to think back to what it was like before I was depressed."

    b. "If I can't explain my point of view in a reasonable way to my buddy, then maybe I should reconsider."

    c. "I should try to look for other options when looking at a situation realistically."

    d. "There is only one correct way to look at a situation. I just have to find that one way."

6. Which of the following statements by a family member of a depressed client indicates that the family member needs further teaching?

    a. "Depression is a result of chemical imbalance."

    b. "Recovery will require a great deal of willpower for my family member."

    c. "Depression is like any medical disorder that needs treatment."

    d. "Depression can happen at any age."

7. A mother of a depressed adolescent states, "I just don't understand the diagnosis. My son has never complained of feeling sad. Sure his grades are getting worse and he has a lot of headaches, but all kids go through that." What characteristics would it be important to emphasize with the mother?

    a. Depression in adolescence does not always look the same as adult depression.

    b. Adolescent boys are more likely to cover up depression than any other age-group.

    c. The headaches he is experiencing do not have a relationship to his depression.

    d. His grades are likely a result of his headaches.

8. A client with depression has the following symptoms: depressed mood most every day, lack of interest in hobbies, loss of weight, high blood pressure, increased white blood cell count, low heart rate, inability to sleep through the night, and loss of energy. How many of these symptoms are associated with depression?

    a. Three

    b. Four

    c. Five

    d. Six

9. An older adult is being examined. Which symptom detected by the advanced-practice psychiatric nurse would indicate that the client is experiencing dementia instead of depression?

    a. The client's forgetfulness fluctuates.

    b. The client can state where she is.

    c. The onset of symptoms has taken place over a long period of time.

    d. The client recognizes that she is in need of help.

10. Which of the following interventions should the nurse include in the implementation phase of the nursing process for a client who is depressed?

    a. Allow the client time alone to process therapy sessions

    b. Provide psychotherapeutic education once the client responds to the medications

    c. Provide activities by which the client will be challenged

    d. Maintain a safe environment

—NOTES—

CHAPTER 10

The Client with a Bipolar Disorder

This chapter presents the spectrum of bipolar disorder, cultural considerations, and the causative factors or theories surrounding bipolar disorder. Various treatment modalities are addressed, as well as treatment considerations, especially psychosocial and behavioral aspects.

Reading Assignment

Prior to beginning this assignment, please read Chapter 10, "The Client with a Bipolar Disorder."

Activities

Using the content in the text, answer the following question as clearly as you can and in your own words. Give examples, if appropriate, to help clarify the information in your answer.

1. Explain the major differences between bipolar I and bipolar II disorders. (p. 269)

_____

_____

_____

_____

_____

Case Study

Suggested answers for Case Studies are provided in the Answers section at the back of this Study Guide.

Scenario:
The new overnight client admission is awake and pacing the halls as the day shift arrives for work. The night report states the client has not slept since arriving at 2300 and that the family states the client has been up for several days yelling and threatening to "make things right." On the unit the client is loud and demanding and attempts to make jokes that are offensive. The client tells about being the marshal at a famous holiday parade and of winning a major

national honor for elementary teachers. When asked what brought her into the hospital, the client states, "It is jealousy. The other teachers can't stand it that I am Teacher of the Year. I just don't understand why they get so mad when I change their test questions. They certainly need the help. You would think they would be grateful. Instead they put me in here!" When asked about her health history, the client responds with a long, drawn-out monologue that rarely addresses her health but rather rambles on about others and how they have treated her.

1. What are the key symptoms that support the diagnosis of bipolar disorder?

    _____
    _____
    _____
    _____
    _____

2. What are additional assessment questions that should be asked?

    _____
    _____
    _____
    _____
    _____

3. What is the primary nursing diagnosis?

    _____
    _____
    _____
    _____
    _____

4. What are some other nursing diagnoses that should be considered for this client?

    _____
    _____
    _____
    _____
    _____

5. What will likely be included in the treatment of this client?

    _____
    _____
    _____
    _____
    _____

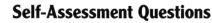

Self-Assessment Questions

Answers and rationales for Self-Assessment Questions are provided in the Answers section at the back of this Study Guide.

1. Which of the following clients is most likely to be diagnosed with bipolar I disorder?

   a. Recent admission data indicate a manic episode with racing thoughts, poor judgment, and inability to sleep.

   b. A client has had numerous depressive and manic episodes, and his mother and grandfather have the same diagnosis.

   c. The history of a community mental health client indicates a high energy level with unusual artistic abilities. The client has remained employed as a waitress.

   d. An inpatient client upon admission complains of hearing voices and seeing "arms coming out of the walls."

2. When teaching a newly diagnosed client with a bipolar disorder, it is important to include which of the following concepts?

   a. The development of bipolar disorder occurs randomly and apparently has no genetic basis.

   b. Bipolar disorder runs in families because children "learn" the behaviors that are present in close family members.

   c. Biological and genetic factors may be the most likely factors in the development of a bipolar disorder.

   d. The most common factor is a brain injury or trauma experienced at an early age, resulting in a brain lesion.

3. Which description of symptoms is most closely associated with a child with manic behavior?

   a. Sudden outbursts several times per day

   b. Inordinate happiness and cheer lasting several days at a time

   c. Unusual level of energy focused on a single task until completed

   d. Elevated mood once or twice per month

4. The use of lithium as a mood stabilizer is prescribed because:

   a. Lithium is the only known pharmacologic agent that is effective for bipolar disorder.

   b. Lithium can be used as only a temporary pharmacologic treatment because of the risk of addiction and tolerance.

   c. Lithium can be used only once manic behaviors are in remission.

   d. Lithium is used for both treatment and prevention of mania.

5. A new client admission has the following symptoms: has had insomnia for 5 days, sees "devils walking across the room," cannot recall when she ate last, carries a large notebook with numerous unusual drawings and lists of projects that are in "the works," and has drawn abstract pictures in ink on her forearms and clothing. The client has threatened to stab her neighbor. The client is diagnosed with bipolar I, severe with psychotic features. What nursing diagnosis is of highest priority?

   a. Disturbed body image

   b. Impaired social interaction

   c. Impaired swallowing

   d. Risk for violence

6. A new client admission has the following symptoms: has had insomnia for 5 days, sees "devils walking across the room," cannot recall when she ate last, carries a large notebook with numerous unusual drawings and lists of projects that are in "the works," and has drawn abstract pictures in ink on her forearms and clothing. The client has threatened to stab her neighbor. The client is diagnosed with bipolar I, severe with psychotic features. The client is prescribed an antipsychotic and an anticonvulsant. The rationale for these two drugs is:

   a. The client also has a form of epilepsy.

   b. The client also has a diagnosis of schizophrenia.

   c. Antipsychotic medications are used as an adjunct to mood stabilizers.

   d. The client is likely allergic to the drug of choice, lithium.

7. A rapidly cycling client with bipolar disorder is being evaluated for medication. The client's chief complaint is the "terrible depression I have several times a year." Which medication is least likely to be prescribed for this client?

   a. An antidepressant

   b. An antipsychotic

   c. Lithium

   d. An anticonvulsant

8. Which statement by a client with a bipolar disorder would indicate that further teaching is needed?

   a. "My family and I need to work on this disease together."

   b. "I should limit my volunteer work to only one or two activities."

   c. "I can keep my job with rotating shifts."

   d. "I need to recognize when I begin to get down on myself."

9. A client with bipolar disorder states in a loud voice, "I really need to get out of the hospital. You know the governor has selected me for Citizen of the Year. I need to get to the award ceremony now!" The nurse's best response is:

   a. "You are not the Citizen of the Year."

   b. "Tell me more about being Citizen of the Year."

   c. "Let's get you some medication."

   d. "I'd like to talk to you a bit more."

10. A client admitted to an acute inpatient psychiatric unit 10 days ago for bipolar disorder eats finger foods while pacing the halls if offered by staff members, draws abstract art in ink on his left hand, sleeps 6 hours each night, and readily takes prescribed medications. Which datum most indicates that the client's condition is improving?

    a. Eats finger foods

    b. Has decreased the amount of "body art"

    c. Sleeps 6 hours

    d. Takes medication

CHAPTER 11

The Client with an Anxiety Disorder

This chapter exposes the student to anxiety across the life span and the various causative factors discussed in this chapter. A nursing process approach is used to plan the care for the client with an anxiety disorder.

Reading Assignment

Prior to beginning this assignment, please read Chapter 11, "The Client with an Anxiety Disorder."

Case Study

Suggested answers for Case Studies are provided in the Answers section at the back of this Study Guide.

Scenario:
A client presents at the emergency department gasping for breath, saying, "I think I am going to die!" On assessment, the heart rate is elevated and the client is diaphoretic. He says he cannot catch his breath and he feels disoriented. He is afraid he will faint at any second. He is tested for cardiac symptoms, and the tests are all negative. When told he has had a panic attack, he refuses to believe it.

1. What symptoms are consistent with panic attack?

    _____

    _____

    _____

    _____

    _____

2. What is the treatment of choice for clients with panic attack?

    _____

    _____

_____

_____

_____

3. What would be important to include in the discharge teaching for this client?

_____

_____

_____

_____

_____

Self-Assessment Questions

Answers and rationales for Self-Assessment Questions are provided in the Answers section at the back of this Study Guide.

1. The nursing assessment indicates that a young child has mild anxiety when performing at a piano recital. Analysis of this finding is:
    a. The child will not be able to remember the music.
    b. The child's anxiety will be transferred to the mother.
    c. The anxiety is detrimental for the child and the performance should be canceled.
    d. The anxiety is conducive to concentration and may improve her performance.

2. A client at the community mental health clinic brings a sterile towel and places it on any surface on which he sits. Such behavior primarily allows the client to:
    a. Punish himself for being phobic
    b. Receive extra attention for his condition
    c. Reduce his anxiety level
    d. Replace feelings of guilt

3. In teaching the client who must sit on a sterile towel to avoid "germs," the nurse should describe the psychodynamics of the behavior in which of the following ways?
    a. Even though the behavior is unusual, it serves to reduce feelings of anxiety.
    b. The phobic behavior is related to stress in the marriage.
    c. The client is likely hearing voices telling him to behave in this manner.
    d. The client has feelings of inferiority and needs to behave this way as a form of punishment.

4. A priority goal for a client with severe anxiety is that the client will:
    a. Discuss feelings of anxiety within 1 week
    b. Establish contact with reality by the end of the day
    c. Cause no harm to self or others at any time
    d. State three activities to control his own behavior

5. A client who worked at a convenience store was recently robbed, beaten, and left for dead. Upon admission, she states that she cannot sleep because every time she closes her eyes, she sees the robber's boots coming toward her face. She admits feigning death to get the robber to stop kicking her. She is diagnosed with acute stress disorder. What behavioral manifestation will the client likely display?

   a. Confusion

   b. Hallucinations

   c. Difficulty in motor coordination

   d. Constant scanning of the environment

6. When working with a client diagnosed with posttraumatic stress disorder, what is the priority nursing diagnosis?

   a. Fear

   b. Sleep pattern disturbance

   c. Powerlessness

   d. Ineffective coping

7. A client with generalized anxiety disorder is most likely to have a co-occuring psychiatric diagnosis of:

   a. Major depression

   b. Posttraumatic stress disorder

   c. Substance use disorder

   d. Schizophrenia

8. In teaching a client the action of the anxiolytic medication that has been prescribed, it is important to include which of the following concepts?

   a. Gamma-aminobutyric acid (GABA) makes target neurons less sensitive to stimulation.

   b. Increased norepinephrine causes the synaptic gap to be less excitable.

   c. Blocking the reuptake of serotonin increases the excitability of inhibitory neurons.

   d. Monoamine oxidase is stimulated.

9. Which of the following would be the most appropriate goal for a client who has been diagnosed as having social phobia?

   a. The client will describe the trauma she has experienced.

   b. The client will not experience disabling fear of public performance.

   c. The client will avoid the object of phobia.

   d. The client will decrease participation in ritualistic behavior.

10. A client seeks help for a specific phobia, fear of flying. Treatment is systematic desensitization. Which of the following concepts are important to teach this client?

   a. "You will be gradually exposed to various stages of flying while learning to relax."

   b. "You will learn to visualize yourself flying a plane. "

   c. "You will be taught to change your beliefs about flying."

   d. "You will be given medication to make you less sensitive to the anxiety about flying."

—NOTES—

CHAPTER 12

The Client with a Somatization Disorder

Somatization disorders presented in this chapter range from the more commonly associated ones of conversion disorder to the newer classifications of chronic fatigue syndrome and fibromyalgia syndrome. This chapter also presents the cultural context as it relates to somatization disorders, and the psychiatric nurse is encouraged to view the impact of the client's culture on the symptoms that are presented.

Reading Assignment

Prior to beginning this assignment, please read Chapter 12, "The Client with a Somatization Disorder."

Activities

Using the content in the text, answer the following questions as clearly as you can and in your own words. Give examples, if appropriate, to help clarify the information in your answer.

1. Explain the following causative theories related to somatization disorders.

   a. Psychodynamic theories (p. 345)

   _____

   _____

   _____

   _____

   _____

   b. Psychosocial and stress factors (pp. 345–346)

   _____

   _____

   _____

   _____

   _____

c.   Attachment theory (p. 346)

_____

_____

_____

_____

_____

d.   Cognitive-behavioral theories (p. 346)

_____

_____

_____

_____

_____

e.   Neurobiological theories (pp. 346–347)

_____

_____

_____

_____

_____

2.   Identify the symptoms that are expressed within the listed cultures as presented in Table 12–1. (p. 348)

Cultural Expression of Somatization

Culture	Symptoms
West African	_____
	_____
Japanese	_____
	_____
	_____
	_____
Indian	_____
	_____

3.   Fill in the correct information. (pp. 349–355)

Disorder	Prevalence	Core Symptoms	Treatment Modalities
Somatization disorder			
Conversion disorder			
Pain disorder			
Fibromyalgia			

Disorder	Prevalence	Core Symptoms	Treatment Modalities
Hypochrondriasis			
Body dysmorphic disorder			
Chronic fatigue syndrome			

4. Discuss somatoform disorders across the life span as they are seen in each of the following age-groups. (pp. 355–356)

Childhood

_____

_____

_____

_____

_____

Adolescence

_____

_____

_____

_____

_____

Adulthood

_____

_____

_____

_____

_____

Older Adulthood

_____

_____

_____

_____

_____

Case Study

Suggested answers for Case Studies are provided in the Answers section at the back of this Study Guide.

Scenario:
A client was transferred to the psychiatric floor after spending 2 weeks on the neurology floor. She was first admitted for partial paralysis to the lower extremities that started shortly after her husband had died. The couple had been married for 43 years and had no children. After the transfer, she was sobbing quietly in bed when the nursing student entered the room and sat near the bed. By using active listening and therapeutic verbal and nonverbal communication, the student learned that the client was experiencing extreme guilt over her husband's death 6 months earlier.

1. Paralysis related to guilt is associated with what somatization disorder?

   _____

   _____

   _____

   _____

   _____

2. What approach is most effective for interacting with this client?

   _____

   _____

   _____

   _____

   _____

3. What is the expected prognosis?

   _____

   _____

   _____

   _____

   _____

Self-Assessment Questions

Answers and rationales for Self-Assessment Questions are provided in the Answers section at the back of this Study Guide.

1. A client develops a paralysis in both legs following the death of her husband. During therapy for conversion reaction, the client describes overwhelming guilt over the choices she made regarding his treatment options prior to his death. Which of the following behaviors observed by the nurse would be an example of primary gain?

   a. Relief from feelings of anxiety

   b. Sympathy for her from friends and family members

   c. Neighbors bringing food items to her home

   d. Indifference to the paralysis that she is experiencing

2. A client develops a paralysis in both legs following the death of her husband. During therapy for conversion reaction, the client describes overwhelming guilt over the choices she made regarding his treatment options prior to his death. What nursing diagnosis is most appropriate for this client?

    a.   Powerlessness

    b.   Ineffective coping

    c.   Social isolation

    d.   Self-care deficit

3. A client develops a paralysis in both legs following the death of her husband. During therapy for conversion reaction, the client describes overwhelming guilt over the choices she made regarding his treatment options prior to his death. With therapy the client has made progress and is ready for discharge. Which comment by the client would indicate that nursing interventions have been successful?

    a.   "I understand now why the neighbors have been so helpful to me."

    b.   "I notice that my legs feel their weakest when I remember what it was like that day in the emergency room."

    c.   "I am done talking about all this. I came here to learn to re-walk again."

    d.   "I'll be fine as long as I rest every day and relax."

4. A client with fibromyalgia has just been diagnosed. In teaching this client about the condition, it is important for the nurse to include which of the following concepts?

    a.   "The pain that you feel will remain localized to the area it is felt now."

    b.   "The pain that you feel will be limited to 4 to 5 sites maximum."

    c.   "Your pain will likely cause you to sleep more hours than normal."

    d.   "Depression is a common problem with your condition."

5. During individual psychotherapy with a client with hypochondriasis, the advanced-practice nurse is asked by the client, "You do believe when I say I am very sick, don't you?" The nurse's most appropriate response is:

    a.   "I believe you are experiencing the symptoms that you describe."

    b.   "I know you think you are, but in reality you do not have these symptoms."

    c.   "I think you are malingering."

    d.   "I believe your symptoms will go away with the proper medical interventions."

6. Which statement by the client with hypchondriasis would indicate an understanding of the disorder?

    a.   "I know my condition is rare, so it is hard for the doctors to confirm my illness with typical lab tests."

    b.   "My situation is one that I will just have to learn to live with."

    c.   "I will probably need to take medication for the rest of my life."

    d.   "Even though I am still a little bit worried, I realize there isn't anything seriously wrong with me."

7. The most appropriate nursing diagnosis for a client with chronic pain who rarely leaves her bed except to use the restroom and eat is:

   a. Impaired role performance

   b. Fear

   c. Risk for violence, self-directed

   d. Powerlessness

8. A client with body dysmorphic disorder has had several plastic surgeries to reshape his nose. The client states, "I am embarrassed to go out in public because everyone stares at my huge nose. Why can't the surgeon get it right?" The most appropriate nursing diagnosis is:

   a. Situational low self-esteem

   b. Anxiety

   c. Disturbed body image

   d. Knowledge deficit

9. A client is determined to malinger. What behavior will the client most likely exhibit?

   a. Vague descriptions of physical ailments

   b. Manipulative behaviors

   c. Overt anxiety

   d. Guilty feelings

CHAPTER 13

The Client with a Stress-Related Disorder

Stress-related disorders are prevalent in today's society. This chapter addresses them in terms of causal relationships and various treatment modalities. Much emphasis is placed on the effects of stress on various organs, with a look at the resulting disease processes.

Reading Assignment

Prior to beginning this assignment, please read Chapter 13, "The Client with a Stress-Related Disorder."

Activities

Using the content in the text, answer the following questions as clearly as you can and in your own words. Give examples, as appropriate, to help clarify the information in your answer.

1. Explain the following causative theories related to stress-related disorders. (pp. 367–371)

   Psychodynamic theory

   _____

   _____

   _____

   _____

   _____

   Neurobiological theory

   _____

   _____

   _____

   _____

   _____

Cognitive and behavioral theories

_____

_____

_____

_____

_____

2. List some of the behaviors that are indicative of Type A personalities. (p. 368)

a. _____

b. _____

c. _____

d. _____

e. _____

f. _____

g. _____

3. List the short-term effects of stress on various organs of the body. (Figure 13–1, pp. 369–370)

Physical and Emotional Effects of Stress

Organ Affected	Short-term Effects

4. List four therapeutic measures that are used for stress-related illness and the indications for their use. (Table 13–2, p. 373)

a. _____

b. _____

c. _____

d. _____

5. Fill in the correct information from Table 13–3. (p. 376)

Specific Psychophysiological Disorders

System	Disorders/Symptoms
Cardiovascular	
Pulmonary	
Immunological	
Gastrointestinal	
Dermatological	
Endocrine	

Case Study

Suggested answers for Case Studies are provided in the Answers section at the back of this Study Guide.

Scenario:
A client with a recent diagnosis of hypertension is referred to the mental health clinic for additional treatment. At the time of the referral, the client's blood pressure is normal, but only with medications.

1. What benefit might the mental health clinic provide to the client?

    _____

    _____

    _____

    _____

    _____

2. What nursing diagnosis might be considered for this client?

    _____

    _____

    _____

    _____

    _____

3. What assessment areas must be covered during the initial interview with this client?

    _____

    _____

    _____

    _____

    _____

Self-Assessment Questions

Answers and rationales for Self-Assessment Questions are provided in the Answers section at the back of this Study Guide.

1. A client with irritable bowel syndrome has asked the nurse to explain the cause of the disorder. The nurse should include in the teaching which of the following concepts?
    a. The condition is not life-threatening.
    b. The condition is closely associated with hypertension.
    c. Once treatment begins, cure is achieved in a short amount of time.
    d. The disorder is debilitating and affects numerous body systems.

2. In teaching a client with a stress-related disorder, the nurse should include which of the following?
    a. "It is essential that you are able to recognize your feelings."
    b. "You will likely be on medication the rest of your life."
    c. "It is very unlikely that your condition is life-threatening."
    d. "The cause of your condition is unknown."

3. Which statement by a client indicates that further teaching regarding the diagnosis of a stress-related disorder is needed?

   a. "I can use problem-solving skills instead of reacting."

   b. "I am sure lucky I have a Type A personality."

   c. "I am confident that I can achieve my goals."

   d. "It is better to look at the glass as half full than half empty."

4. In teaching a client about biofeedback, the nurse should include which of the following statements?

   a. "You will be hooked up to a machine that measures physical responses."

   b. "You will be taught to change your beliefs about your feelings."

   c. "You will be given medication in conjunction with your therapy."

   d. "You will be gradually exposed to various stages of anxiety while learning to relax."

5. A client has severe symptoms of irritable bowel syndrome. Which nursing diagnosis is most appropriate for this client?

   a. Imbalanced nutrition: less than body requirements

   b. Feeding self-care deficit

   c. Delayed growth and development

   d. Risk for fluid volume deficit

6. The nurses are talking about a client admitted for coronary heart disease. Which statement is most likely to be associated with a person having coronary heart disease?

   a. "No matter what I do, I can't seem to do the right thing for this client."

   b. "I have seldom met someone who is so bashful and shy."

   c. "What a funny guy!"

   d. "He is so laid back and nonjudgmental."

7. A client with asthma asks, "What is causing my symptoms?" The most appropriate response by the nurse is:

   a. "Asthma is caused by stress."

   b. "Asthma is exacerbated by stressful situations."

   c. "Asthma is caused by unmet dependency needs."

   d. "Asthma is an expression of the anger that you feel."

CHAPTER 14

The Client with Schizophrenia and Other Psychotic Disorders

In this chapter, various theories surrounding the nature and causes of schizophrenia are presented. Reference is made to other disorders that may mimic schizophrenia, as well as to the various treatment modalities and approaches, including nursing care for the schizophrenic patient.

Reading Assignment

Prior to beginning this assignment, please read Chapter 14, "The Client with Schizophrenia and Other Psychotic Disorders."

Activities

Using the content in the text, answer the following questions as clearly as you can and in your own words. Give examples, if appropriate, to help clarify the information in your answer.

1. Compare the acute and prodromal phases of the course of schizophrenia using Table 14–2. (p. 388)

Schizophrenia: Course of the Illness

	Acute (Active) Phase	Prodromal and Residual Phases
Definition		
Symptoms		
Minimum duration		

2. List the positive, negative, and cognitive symptoms of schizophrenia. (pp. 394–395)

_____

_____

_____

_____

_____

Case Study

Suggested answers for Case Studies are provided in the Answers section at the back of this Study Guide.

Scenario:

A client is admitted to the high-security unit of the psychiatric facility. On admission he is agitated, stating, "I am not safe here. I am not safe anywhere." He admits to seeing things that no one else sees. He speaks under his breath while pacing the hall. His appearance is unkempt and his behavior is disorganized. He can be observed laughing while staring at the wall. He can often be found curled up in bed or sitting in the corner of the room with his back against the wall. When he is asked a question, he appears not to take notice and remains lost in his own thoughts.

1. What behaviors are associated with the negative symptoms of schizophrenia?

_____

_____

_____

2. What behaviors are associated with the positive symptoms of schizophrenia?

_____

_____

_____

3. What behaviors are associated with cognitive symptoms of schizophrenia?

_____

_____

_____

4. What nursing diagnoses should be considered for this client?

_____

_____

_____

5. What nursing interventions should be employed?

_____

_____

_____

6. What pharmacologic interventions will likely be used?

_____

_____

_____

Self-Assessment Questions

Answers and rationales for Self-Assessment Questions are provided in the Answers section at the back of this Study Guide.

1. Which of the following symptoms is associated with the negative symptoms of schizophrenia?
   a. Seeing the devil's face on the wall
   b. Hearing voices asking the client to jump off a bridge
   c. Client's belief that she can fly
   d. Blunted affect

2. When the nurse scratches her head, the client scratches his head. When the nurse crosses her leg, the client crosses his leg. This is an example of which symptom?
   a. Echolalia
   b. Echopraxia
   c. Imitation
   d. Avolition

3. A psychotic client is heard to say: "I see things that ring so I can sing. What did you bring?" This is an example of:
   a. Word salad
   b. Tangentiality
   c. Concrete thinking
   d. Clang associations

4. During assessment a nurse asks the client where he lives. His response is, "I live in the room with a bed behind the kitchen." This response is typical of which symptom?
   a. Neologism
   b. Circumstantiality
   c. Concrete thinking
   d. Hallucinations

5. A client believes he is the chauffeur for a major movie star. He describes the limousine that is at his disposal and brags about all of the famous people that he has met. What type of delusion is he exhibiting?
   a. Delusion of grandeur
   b. Delusion of persecution
   c. Delusion of reference
   d. Delusion of control

6. A client says, "Watch out! There is someone standing right behind you." There is no one else there. The appropriate response by the nurse is:

    a. "I understand that you see someone, but I don't see anyone there."

    b. "Let's move away to the other room."

    c. "Tell me more about what you see."

    d. "You are not seeing anything."

7. Interventions for the client who is actively hallucinating include:

    a. Touching the client to convey warmth and concern

    b. Teaching the client to tell the voices to go away

    c. Providing a quiet and dimly lit environment without radios or TVs

    d. Allowing the client to rest in his room undisturbed

8. Which of the following clients is most likely diagnosed with catatonic schizophrenia?

    a. A client in a state of stupor who is unresponsive to his surroundings and is mute

    b. A client who believes that the FBI is after him

    c. A client without delusions, hallucinations, confusion, or disorganized thoughts

    d. A client who is confused and whose conversation rambles

9. A client with schizophrenia sees things that no one sees and hears things no one else hears, and his speech rhymes when he speaks. Which of the following nursing diagnosis is most appropriate for this client?

    a. Disturbed thought processes

    b. Disturbed sensory perception

    c. Chronic low self-esteem

    d. Ineffective coping

10. The mother of an adolescent newly diagnosed with schizophrenia asks, "What causes this disorder?" After the teaching is complete, which statement by the mother indicates that further teaching is necessary?

    a. "There may be genetic reason for his disorder."

    b. "There is a chemical in the brain called dopamine that may be elevated."

    c. "Stress caused him to be this way."

    d. "His brain may have some structural differences."

CHAPTER 15

The Client with a Personality Disorder

In this chapter, personality disorders are clustered according to similarities in characteristics. A comparison of these disorders is made according to their characteristics and treatment modalities.

Reading Assignment

Prior to beginning this assignment, please read Chapter 15, "The Client with a Personality Disorder."

Activities

Using the content in the text, answer the following questions as clearly as you can and in your own words. Give examples, if appropriate, to help clarify the information in your answer.

1. Identify healthy and unhealthy ego functions as they relate to personality disorders. (Table 15–3, p. 418)

Comparison of Healthy and Unhealthy Ego Functions

	Healthy Ego Functions (Mature)	Unhealthy Ego Functions (Primitive)
Defense mechanisms		
Modulation of affect		
Self-esteem		
Relationship to others		
Reality testing		
Cognitive processes		

2. Identify the maladaptive behaviors that may be exhibited across the life span and associated possible causes. (Table 15–4, p. 419)

Maladaptive Coping Behaviors Arising in Early Developmental Periods and Continuing across the Life Span

	Maladaptive Behavior	**Possible Cause**
Infancy		
Childhood		
Adolescence		
Early and middle adulthood		
Older adulthood		

3. List the causes and characteristics of conduct disorder. (Table 15–5, p. 424)

Causes and Characteristics of Conduct Disorder

	Causes	**Characteristics**
Psychological		
Neurobiological		
Sociological		

4. Compare the symptoms of schizoid and schizotypal disorders. (Table 15–6, p. 430)

Symptoms of Schizoid and Schizotypal Disorders

Schizoid Disorders	**Schizotypal Disorders**
1.	1.
2.	2.
3.	3.
4.	4.
5.	5.
6.	6.
7.	7.
	8.
	9.

5. The nursing interventions that are appropriate for clients who are diagnosed with schizotypal and schizoid personality disorders are: (p. 430)

a. _____

b. _____

c. _____

d. _____

e. _____

f. _____

6. List the characteristics of the diagnoses that make up Cluster II personality disorders. (pp. 430–432)

Characteristics of Cluster II Personality Disorders

Antisocial	Borderline Personality Disorder	Histrionic	Narcissistic

Case Study

Suggested answers for Case Studies are provided in the Answers section at the back of this Study Guide.

Scenario:
A client is readmitted for the fourth time this year, having made a suicide attempt. The client complains that she is bored with life and has nothing to live for. She recently broke up with her boyfriend of 6 weeks, stating, "I really thought he was going to be the one. We fell madly, passionately in love at first sight, but it only lasted 2 weeks. After that we fought all the time." She has numerous scars on her wrists and forearms.

1. What personality disorder should be considered for this client?

_____

_____

_____

_____

_____

2. What is the theoretical foundation for this disorder?

_____

_____

_____

_____

_____

3. What nursing diagnosis should be considered?

_____

_____

_____

_____

4. What treatment options are available?

_____

_____

_____

_____

_____

Self-Assessment Questions

Answers and rationales for Self-Assessment Questions are provided in the Answers section at the back of this Study Guide.

1. A client is diagnosed with a personality disorder. The primary behaviors the client exhibits are odd behavior and appearance with unusually colored hair, lack of friends, comments that he believes black birds flying overhead are a bad omen, and an aloof manner. These behaviors are most closely associated with which personality disorder?

   a. Narcissistic

   b. Avoidant

   c. Passive-aggressive

   d. Schizotypal

2. An advanced-practice psychiatric nurse works on boundaries with clients who have a borderline personality disorder. An accurate description of this is:

   a. Clients will be limited in where they can live due to the severity of their symptoms.

   b. Clients will be encouraged to reflect and act upon their most basic feelings.

   c. The nurse teaches what are maladaptive behaviors, and when observed, consequences are enforced.

   d. Clear rules are defined for who and how members participate in a relationship.

3. An adolescent is diagnosed with conduct disorder. Which of the following behaviors is likely present?

   a. Arguing with parents

   b. Being cruel to animals

   c. Teasing siblings

   d. Temper tantrums

4. A co-worker makes the following statements about conduct disorders. Which statement indicates the co-worker needs further teaching about conduct disorders?

   a. "The prognosis for the adolescent with conduct disorder is very good."

   b. "I see more boys with this disorder than girls."

   c. "Temperament can have something to do with the cause of conduct disorders."

   d. "Skipping school is very common in clients with conduct disorder."

5. Which of the following behaviors is likely seen in a child with oppositional defiant disorder?
   a. Setting a fire in the garage to watch it burn
   b. Engaging in sexual activity at an early age
   c. Stealing jewelry from his mother
   d. Leaving the garbage in the house when he is expected to take it out

6. A client with a personality disorder is prescribed an antipsychotic medication. Of the following choices, which type of personality disorder is the client most likely to have?
   a. Schizoid
   b. Antisocial
   c. Passive-aggressive
   d. Histrionic

7. A nurse gathers the following data during the assessment of a client. The client brags about famous people that he knows. He relates that he daydreams about how successful he can be. He states that he is too good to be rooming with the client in the next bed. Which personality disorder is indicated by this behavior?
   a. Histrionic
   b. Narcissistic
   c. Antisocial
   d. Avoidant

8. Which nursing intervention should be employed with a client who has a borderline personality disorder?
   a. "I see you have made your bed today and cleaned up your room."
   b. "I have a few minutes. Would you like to play a game of cards?"
   c. "Your roommate is looking to play scrabble. I think he would enjoy it if you joined him."
   d. "I plan to meet with you every day at 10 a.m. when I am working."

9. Which response by the nurse is inappropriate when working with a client who has a nursing diagnosis of disturbed personal identity?
   a. "I know you are feeling upset."
   b. "Tell me more about that feeling."
   c. "I am having trouble understanding that."
   d. "I am interested in hearing more about that."

10. A client with borderline personality disorder has been admitted after cutting her arms deeply. The wounds need a dressing change. The nurse should change the dressing in the following manner:
    a. Provide genuine concern for the pain she is feeling at the wound site
    b. At the client's request, add an extra but unnecessary large bandage to the area
    c. Ask her to reflect on her feelings concerning the need to have someone change her dressings
    d. Use a nonjudgmental approach without commenting on the wound

—NOTES—

CHAPTER 16

The Client with Delirium, Dementia, Amnestic, and Other Cognitive Disorders

Dementia, delirium, amnestic, and other cognitive disorders are discussed in this chapter. As with the other chapters on psychiatric disorders, the nursing process approach is used to assist the psychiatric nurse in planning and implementing care for these challenging disorders.

Reading Assignment

Prior to beginning this assignment, please read Chapter 16, "The Client with Delirium, Dementia, Amnestic, and Other Cognitive Disorders."

Activities

Using the content in the text, answer the following questions as clearly as you can and in your own words. Give examples, if appropriate, to help clarify the information in your answer.

1. List the developmental changes with age. (Table 16–1, p. 460)

Stage/Age	Change Noted

2. List the factors that are associated with the development of delirium. (Table 16–2, p. 462)

Category

Factor

_____ _____
_____ _____
_____ _____
_____ _____
_____ _____
_____ _____
_____ _____
_____ _____

3. Identify the commonly used drugs that can cause delirium. (Table 16–3, p. 463)

Commonly Used Drugs Causing Delirium

Group	Example(s)

4. Discuss causes of mental retardation. (Table 16–4, p. 465)

Genetic

Acquired

_____ _____
_____ _____
_____ _____
_____ _____
_____ _____
_____ _____
_____ _____
_____ _____
_____ _____
_____ _____
_____ _____

5. Using the table below, indicate the areas that are affected and the patterns of malformation related to fetal alcohol syndrome. (Table 16–5, p. 466)

Fetal Alcohol Syndrome: Patterns of Malformation

Affected Area	Pattern of Malformation

6. List the stages of Alzheimer's disease. (Table 16–6, p. 469)

a. _____

b. _____

c. _____

d. _____

7. Identify several guidelines that should be used in caring for a client with a cognitive disorder. (p. 478)

• _____
_____
_____

• _____
_____
_____

• _____
_____
_____

• _____
_____
_____

• _____
_____
_____

8. In relation to the interventions that may be used for persons with cognitive disorders, list some activities related to each intervention. (pp. 482–483)

Intervention	Activities
Delirium management	_____ _____
Dementia management	_____ _____
Limit setting	_____ _____
Medication management	_____ _____

Case Study

Suggested answers for Case Studies are provided in the Answers section at the back of this Study Guide.

Scenario:
An elderly woman's family is concerned about her failing memory. They have brought their mother into the clinic for a comprehensive evaluation.

1. What assessment activities are important to conduct to determine the woman's cognitive functioning?

    _____

    _____

    _____

2. What options should the family consider in determining whether the mother can remain in her own home or whether alternative living arrangements should be made?

    _____

    _____

    _____

3. If the diagnosis should be Alzheimer's disease, what prognosis is likely?

    _____

    _____

    _____

4. What pharmacologic intervention would be considered for her if Alzheimer's were confirmed?

    _____

    _____

    _____

Self-Assessment Questions

Answers and rationales for Self-Assessment Questions are provided in the Answers section at the back of this Study Guide.

1. A daughter calls the community health clinic and states that her mother can no longer balance her checkbook. She asks whether she should be concerned about her mother's behavior. The nurse identifies this behavior as which of the following symptoms associated with dementia?
    a.   Abulia
    b.   Acalculia
    c.   Anomia
    d.   Apraxic agraphia

2. A nursing home resident on an Alzheimer's unit picks up a fork and is unable to identify it. This is an example of which of the following symptoms?
    a.   Abulia
    b.   Acalculia
    c.   Anomia
    d.   Apraxia

3. A son visits his mother at Christmas. The last time he visited her home was on Mother's Day weekend. In May, he noticed that she was forgetful but saw no cause for concern. Now at Christmas he discovers she has been using her bathtub as her toilet. This behavior is an example of which of the following symptoms?
    a.   Chorea
    b.   Apraxia
    c.   Asimultanagnosia
    d.   Alogia

4. A client is asked to copy a simple geometric shape as part of the assessment for dementia. The client is unable to do so. The purpose of this assessment technique is to determine whether the client has:
    a.   Apraxic agraphia
    b.   Constructional praxis
    c.   Asimultanagnosia
    d.   Semantic paraphasia

5. Which of the following conditions is characterized as delirium?
    a.   A gradual increase in using the word "thing" for most objects when conversing
    b.   Sudden confusion related to an infection
    c.   Constant jerking and rapid, well-coordinated movements
    d.   An insidious course of confusion and forgetfulness

6. Which of the following comments by the daughter of a recently diagnosed client with Alzheimer's requires further teaching?

   a.   "With treatment, my mother should soon show improvement."

   b.   " I will need to find assisted living arrangements for my mother."

   c.   "At some point, she will be unable to walk."

   d.   "Forgetfulness is just the beginning of what we can expect."

7. A confused client is sitting at the breakfast table but is not eating. The most appropriate comment by the nurse is:

   a.   "Take a bite of this food."

   b.   "Mrs. S, it is 7 a.m. Time for breakfast."

   c.   "I know you are going to love what the cook has fixed today."

   d.   "What was your favorite food when you were younger?"

8. A client is admitted to the intensive care unit with multiple injuries following a car accident. The client's drug screen is positive for methamphetamine. Which of the following interventions is counterproductive while the client is still under the influence of the methamphetamine?

   a.   Say, "You are safe here in the hospital."

   b.   Say, "This is a machine that will help you to breathe."

   c.   Keep the lights bright to reduce shadows.

   d.   Limit visitation.

9. A client with dementia gets out of bed in the middle of the night. He is quite agitated and keeps saying, "Where is the barn? I got to get them cows milked or they will dry up." The nurse's best response is:

   a.   "It is OK. I already milked the cows, you can go back to bed."

   b.   "There are no cows to milk."

   c.   "Here is your medication."

   d.   "The cows have already been taken care of."

10.   The nursing assistant in a long-term care facility complains that a client with dementia is constantly incontinent. The nurse should instruct the nursing assistant to:

   a.   Provide frequent and thorough skin care

   b.   Include an adult diaper product as part of the client's hygiene each morning

   c.   Take the client into the bathroom every 2 to 3 hours and sit the client on the toilet

   d.   Teach the client to use a hand signal to indicate he needs to use the toilet

CHAPTER 17

The Client with Attention-Deficit Disorder

This chapter presents the causative factors and the historical perspectives related to attention-deficit disorder, as well as the symptoms of ADHD that can be seen in individuals across the life span. The nursing process approach to the care of the patient with ADHD is addressed, with an emphasis on behavioral interventions that are appropriate for individuals with ADHD.

Reading Assignment

Prior to beginning this assignment, please read Chapter 17, "The Client with Attention-Deficit Disorder."

Activities

Using the content in the text, answer the following questions as clearly as you can and in your own words. Give examples, if appropriate, to help clarify the information in your answer.

1. Explain the following causative theories related to attention-deficit disorder. (pp. 497–499)

   Brain injury _____

   _____

   _____

   Dietary intake_____

   _____

   _____

   Environmental toxins_____

   _____

   _____

   Genetics _____

   _____

   _____

Neurobiological basis _____

_____

_____

2. ADHD is often complicated by co-occurring conditions, such as: (p. 508)

    a. _____

    b. _____

    c. _____

    d. _____

3. List way in which psychoeducation may be effective in the treatment of ADHD. (p. 510)

    • _____

    _____

    • _____

    _____

    • _____

    _____

    • _____

    _____

4. List some of the nursing diagnoses related to the client with ADHD and the associated outcomes. (p. 512)

Nursing Diagnosis	Outcome

5. List some of the medications that may be used in the treatment of ADHD, their target symptoms, and the ways in which they work. (Table 17–4, p. 516)

Medications Used in the Treatment of ADHD

Type	Name	How it Works	Target Symptoms

6. Identify some of the principles that should be used to enhance a behavior management plan. (p. 517)

- _____
- _____
- _____
- _____
- _____
- _____
- _____

Case Study

Suggested answers for Case Studies are provided in the Answers section at the back of this Study Guide.

Scenario:
An 8-year-old child presents with the following symptoms: constant restlessness while awake, short attention span, and impulsive behaviors such as taking other children's belongings and shoplifting. The child is failing school and has few friends. The parents are very concerned but blame each other for poor parenting skills.

1. What key assessment question needs to be determined before a diagnosis of attention-deficit disorder can be considered?

   _____
   _____
   _____

2. What therapy should be considered?

   _____
   _____
   _____

3. What pharmacologic intervention might be prescribed for the child?

   _____
   _____
   _____

Self-Assessment Questions

Answers and rationales for Self-Assessment Questions are provided in the Answers section at the back of this Study Guide.

1. A young client has been referred by the school psychologist to the community mental health clinic for evaluation of possible attention-deficit disorder. The school describes the child's behavior as restless in the classroom and frequently given to temper tantrums. What additional behaviors are consistent with a diagnosis of attention-deficit/hyperactivity disorder?
   a. Poor eating habits
   b. Inability to fall asleep at night
   c. Distractibility
   d. Repetition of meaningless hand signals

2. Which comment by the mother is significant in making the diagnosis of attention-deficit/hyperactivity disorder?

   a. "He has always been full of energy. Even at age four, it was impossible to get him settled down."

   b. "After school, he comes home and plays with his Legos for hours if I let him."

   c. "He still sucks his thumb when he thinks I am not looking."

   d. "He will make his bed if I remind him to do so."

3. Which of the following symptoms of attention deficit is not typical of the adult client?

   a. Numerous jobs within a span of 2 years

   b. High energy and in constant motion

   c. Tools and checkbook frequently misplaced

   d. Marital problems with spouse

4. The nurse expects three of the following interventions for the client with ADHD. Which intervention is not associated with ADHD?

   a. Behavior contract

   b. Antipsychotic medication

   c. Cognitive therapy for the family

   d. Psychostimulant medication

5. The mother of a child newly diagnosed with ADHD calls the nurse at the community mental health clinic. She states she has done some reading on her son's medication and the information says that the drug the son is taking is a stimulant. The mother asks, "How can this be the right drug for my son? I thought he was hyperactive. Won't this medication make him more hyper?" The best response by the nurse is:

   a. "Bring your son into the clinic right away. The doctor will need to see him as soon as possible."

   b. "I am sure that the medication was ordered correctly, but let me call the pharmacy where you had the prescription filled and clarify what happened."

   c. "A stimulant is prescribed because it increases the type of chemicals in the brain that improve focus and concentration."

   d. "The information that you accessed is incorrect."

6. Which statement by a parent of a child with ADHD indicates that further teaching is necessary?

   a. "I will need to give my son his medication once every week, preferably before bedtime."

   b. "The dosage that my son needs will have to be based on how he responds to the medication instead of on how tall he is and how much he weighs."

   c. "I am sure glad that there has been about 50 years of experience treating ADHD with medication."

   d. "My son will need to have lab tests periodically."

7. Three of the following side effects are common with stimulant medication. Identify the side effect that is not associated with stimulant medication.

    a. Insomnia

    b. Increased appetite

    c. Headache

    d. Irritability

8. A young client attends the partial program at a community mental health center that includes treatment for his ADHD and schooling. His behaviors include excessive fidgeting with his pencil, interruption of his peers when they are speaking, getting up from his desk without permission, blurting out answers to the special education teacher's questions without raising his hand, and talking incessantly. What is the most appropriate nursing diagnosis for this client?

    a. Impaired social interactions

    b. Risk for suicide

    c. Panic

    d. Disturbed thought processes

9. A young client attends the partial program at a community mental health center that includes treatment for his ADHD and schooling. His behaviors include excessive fidgeting with his pencil, interruption of his peers when they are speaking, getting up from his desk without permission, blurting out answers to the special education teacher's questions without raising his hand, and talking incessantly. When the client interrupts the teacher, what is the teacher's best response?

    a. "I expect all students to raise their hand to get permission to speak."

    b. "I have told you several times before that you must raise your hand before speaking."

    c. "For speaking out of turn, you will need to stand in the corner of the room."

    d. "Speaking without permission in my classroom is bad."

—NOTES—

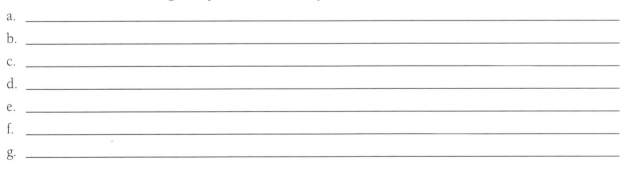

CHAPTER 18

The Client with a Dissociative Disorder

Providing care for clients with a dissociative disorder can prove challenging for the psychiatric nurse. This chapter presents four examples of dissociative disorders with suggested treatments.

Reading Assignment

Prior to beginning this assignment, please read Chapter 18, "The Client with a Dissociative Disorder."

Activities

Using the content in the text, answer the following questions as clearly as you can and in your own words. Give examples, if appropriate, to help clarify the information in your answer.

1. Define dissociation according to Peplau. (Table 18–1, p. 533)

   a. _____

   b. _____

   c. _____

   d. _____

   e. _____

   f. _____

   g. _____

2. Compare the signs and symptoms of dissociative disorders with those of medical or other psychiatric diagnoses. (Table 18–2, p. 536)

Medical and Other Psychiatric Diagnoses with Symptoms Similar to Those of Dissociative Disorders

Dissociative Disorders	Signs and Symptoms	Medical or Other Psychiatric Diagnoses	Signs and Symptoms

3. List the behavioral features that are common in children with dissociative disorders. (p. 538)

   a. _____

   b. _____

   c. _____

   d. _____

   e. _____

4. Compare and contrast the etiologies of the various dissociative disorders. (pp. 540–541)

Disorder	Etiology	Characteristics and Examples
Depersonalization disorder		
Dissociative amnesia		
Dissociative fugue		
Dissociative identity disorder		

5. List the four main interventions that are used with dissociative disorders. (pp. 541–542)

   a. _____

   b. _____

   c. _____

   d. _____

6. What are the four techniques of grounding that should be taught to the client with a dissociative disorder? (p. 542)

   a. _____

   b. _____

   c. _____

   d. _____

Case Study

Suggested answers for Case Studies are provided in the Answers section at the back of this Study Guide.

Scenario:
After the birth of her first child, a 26-year-old client suddenly has no recollection of her life from age 17 to the present. Although she acknowledges that the baby is "cute," she does not recognize the baby as her own and she does not recognize her husband of 5 years. She has clear memories of her life as a teenager up until age 17 and refers to herself as though she were that age. Her parents are interviewed, and it is discovered that the client was raped by several older teens at age 17. The husband denies ever being told of the incident.

1. What theory would explain the causative factor of the amnesia?

   _____

   _____

   _____

2. What psychosocial interventions are available for treatment of this client?

   _____

   _____

   _____

3. Describe the role of the nurse in the client's therapy.

   _____

   _____

   _____

4. What nursing diagnosis should be considered?

   _____

   _____

   _____

Self-Assessment Questions

Answers and rationales for Self-Assessment Questions are provided in the Answers section at the back of this Study Guide.

1. The community mental health clinic has just admitted a client with a dissociative identity disorder. A co-worker asks what caused the development of this disorder. The best response to the co-worker's request is:
   a. "The disorder is a form of malingering."
   b. "Another name for the disorder is split personality."
   c. "Clients with this disorder have experienced overwhelming abuse as children."
   d. "Secondary gain is the cause of this disorder."

2. A client has several distinct alters, each named with special roles. For instance, Jane is the alter that talks to authority figures and goes to work. Betty is childlike and enjoys playing with dolls. The goal of therapy for this client is to:

    a. Eliminate all but one personality

    b. Assess the qualities of all the alters and abolish those alters that have negative characteristics

    c. Blend all alters into one

    d. Age-progress the child alter

3. A client is admitted with the following history: He made a sudden and unexpected trip from home. He is found wandering the streets in Las Vegas, calling himself by a different name. When his picture is shown on the local news, his brother-in-law recognizes him as his sister's missing husband. The client's behavior is consistent with:

    a. Dissociative fugue

    b. Malingering

    c. Dissociative identity disorder

    d. Depersonalization disorder

4. A client made a sudden and unexpected trip from home. He is found wandering the streets in Las Vegas, calling himself by a different name. When his picture is shown on the local news, his brother-in-law recognizes him as his sister's missing husband. Which of the following is the most appropriate nursing diagnosis for this client?

    a. Ineffective coping

    b. Disturbed sensory perception

    c. Powerlessness

    d. Disturbed body image

5. A client made a sudden and unexpected trip from home. He is found wandering the streets in Las Vegas, calling himself by a different name. When his picture is shown on the local news, his brother-in-law recognizes him as his sister's missing husband. When the client's wife arrives to see her husband, she asks the nurse, "What caused my husband to leave like that and take on this new identity? Will he ever get better?" The best response by the nurse is:

    a. "The amnesia is typically brief."

    b. "He is likely to have some relapses from time to time."

    c. "He will need to be on medication for the rest of his life."

    d. "His condition is oftentimes associated with too much dopamine, a brain chemical."

CHAPTER 19

The Client at Risk of Suicidal and Self-Destructive Behaviors

This chapter presents the causative factors related to suicide. The role of the nurse in caring for suicidal patients and those with self-destructive behaviors is also addressed using a nursing process approach.

Reading Assignment

Prior to beginning this assignment, please read Chapter 19, "The Client at Risk of Suicidal and Self-Destructive Behaviors."

Activities

Using the content in the text, answer the following questions as clearly as you can and in your own words. Give examples, if appropriate, to help clarify the information in your answer.

1. List four myths about suicide and the facts that dispel them. (p. 555)

Myths	Facts

2. List at least three factors in each category that are indicative of a high risk for suicide. (Table 19–1, p. 555)

Clinical Factors Indicating High Suicide Risk

Category	Factor
Psychological	
Behavioral	
Sociocultural	
Neurobiological	
Major demographic	

3. List the causative factors in suicide. (pp. 557–563)

    a. _____

    b. _____

    c. _____

    d. _____

    e. _____

4. Identify examples of cultural factors that increase the risk for suicide in Hispanic females. (Table 19–2, p. 559)

Cultural Factors Increasing the Risk of Suicide Among Hispanic Females

Family Domain	Developmental Factors	Sociocultural Domain	Psychological Domain

5. List some of the questions that nurses may ask clients to explore the reasons behind previous suicide attempts. (p. 564)

    • _____

    • _____

    • _____

    • _____

    • _____

    • _____

    • _____

    • _____

6. Show the prevalence and causative factors of suicide across the life span. (p. 565)

Prevalence and Causative Factors of Suicide across the Life Span

	Prevalence	Causative Factors
Childhood		
Adolescence		
Early/middle adulthood		
Older adulthood		
Total population		

7. List the major concepts to be considered in assessing the suicidal child. (p. 566)

   - _____
   - _____
   - _____
   - _____
   - _____
   - _____
   - _____

8. For the suicidal client, the major nursing interventions should include the following: (p. 575)

   a. _____
   b. _____
   c. _____
   d. _____
   e. _____
   f. _____

9. List the legal considerations in the care of the suicidal client. (Table 19–5, p. 575)

   - _____
   - _____
   - _____
   - _____
   - _____
   - _____

10. What are some of the nursing interventions used in caring for the suicidal client in the least restrictive environment? (p. 575)

    - _____
    - _____
    - _____
    - _____

11. List some nursing diagnoses that may be appropriate for the suicidal client. (p. 576)

    a. _____
    b. _____
    c. _____
    d. _____

12. What are the components of a psychological autopsy? (pp. 578–579)

    - _____
    - _____
    - _____
    - _____

Case Study

Suggested answers for Case Studies are provided in the Answers section at the back of this Study Guide.

Scenario:
An elderly client is admitted with suicidal ideations. The client has recently lost his spouse of 53 years. Although he owns his home, there is little money to pay taxes and repairs. His adult children live several hundreds of miles away and rarely visit. In his younger years, he hunted deer and pheasants. He still has guns in the home. Last month his doctor diagnosed cataracts, and the client has difficulty reading.

1. What assessments must be asked?

   _____
   _____
   _____

2. What risk factors for suicide are present?

   _____
   _____
   _____

3. What nursing diagnosis is a priority for him?

   _____
   _____
   _____

4. What nursing interventions should be implemented?

   _____
   _____
   _____

Self-Assessment Questions

Answers and rationales for Self-Assessment Questions are provided in the Answers section at the back of this Study Guide.

1. A nurse is working with a suicidal client. Which comment by the nurse is most appropriate?
   a. "To get your mind off of your problems, let's play some cards."
   b. "It will be helpful if you can keep yourself busy."
   c. "Are you having suicidal thoughts at this time?"
   d. "What are your discharge plans?"

2. A suicidal client has shown improvement in his affect today over yesterday. The nurse should:
   a. Continue suicide precautions
   b. Reevaluate the goals of therapy
   c. Focus on the second-highest nursing diagnosis
   d. Make plans for discharge

3. Which of the following individuals would likely have the highest risk for suicide?

    a.   African American female with two children who is going through a divorce

    b.   Unemployed European American male with alcoholism

    c.   Struggling college student

    d.   Teenager living in a single-parent home

4. A new admission to the psychiatric unit was being oriented to the inpatient program. The client was brought into the hospital after his wife found him in the garage, lying on the floor with the car running. Which statement by the client indicates a high risk for suicide?

    a.   "How long do you think I will be in here?"

    b.   "Can I sit out here in the dayroom?"

    c.   "How often do the night nurses come around?"

    d.   "What am I supposed to do all day?"

5. Which of the following is the primary goal for a client who is suicidal?

    a.   The client will make a contract not to harm self.

    b.   The client will seek out staff to talk about feelings.

    c.   The client will express anger.

    d.   The client will verbalize no thoughts of suicide.

6. Which assessment data would be associated with the highest risk of suicide?

    a.   Client has a specific plan to use the gun in the basement by putting the barrel in his mouth and pulling the trigger.

    b.   Client will take a large amount of pills purchased at the pharmacy when things "get too bad."

    c.   Client's parents have found a knotted cord in the garage.

    d.   Client states, "At some point, I will get myself to the river and jump in."

7. Which question by the nurse is the most appropriate to assess for suicide ideation?

    a.   "Are you having thoughts about killing yourself?"

    b.   "Have you ever harmed yourself?"

    c.   "Has anyone in your family hurt themselves?"

    d.   "What do you think about when you are very sad?"

8. A client with borderline personality disorder has made numerous suicidal gestures, mostly of superficial scratches on her forearm. The client has been readmitted for the fourth time this year with suicidal ideation. The nurse should:

    a.   Give as little attention as possible to the client's attention-seeking behavior

    b.   Recognize that the impulsivity of borderline personality disorder makes suicide a very high risk

    c.   Know that the support of the client's multiple close friends will modulate the risk for suicide

    d.   Determine that previous gestures can predict future behavior

9. The mother of a teenage girl calls the community mental health clinic and states, "I know I shouldn't have, but I read my daughter's diary. My daughter is writing about how she plans to drive her car off a cliff. What should I do?" The best response by the nurse is:

    a. "Most teenagers exaggerate and are dramatic, especially when they think no one will know about their thoughts."

    b. "This is normal behavior."

    c. "Teenagers who talk about suicide don't follow through with it. It is the ones who don't that are more at risk."

    d. "Your daughter's behavior may mean she is making serious plans for suicide, and she should be evaluated immediately."

10. A nursing home resident is being visited by her spouse of 53 years. The nurse hears the visitor state, "I just don't think I can go on any longer." The best response by the nurse is:

    a. "I know it is difficult, but your wife needs the care that we can provide."

    b. "At least you still have each other."

    c. "You can't go on any longer?"

    d. "Let me get you a cup of coffee and talk about your wife's care."

CHAPTER 20

The Client Exhibiting Aggression, Hostility, and Violence

This chapter provides a comprehensive review of the theories of violent behaviors and the role of the nurse when working with clients exhibiting aggression, hostility, and violence.

Reading Assignments

Prior to beginning this assignment, please read Chapter 20, "The Client Exhibiting Aggression, Hostility, and Violence."

Activities

Using the content in the text, answer the following questions as clearly as you can and in your own words. Give examples to help clarify the information in your answer.

1. Define agitation, aggression, hostility, and violence. (p. 589)

   _____

   _____

   _____

2. List causative factors associated with violence. (pp. 590–594)

   _____

   _____

   _____

3. Review the nurse-client dialogue box using de-escalation techniques. (p. 595)

   _____

   _____

   _____

4. Discuss individual characteristics associated with violence. (Box 20–2, p. 596)

_____

_____

_____

5. Discuss de-escalation personal safety skills. (Box 20–3, p. 597)

_____

_____

_____

6. Describe the assessment of the client with the potential/actual violence, aggression, and hostility. (p. 600)

_____

_____

_____

7. Discuss pharmacological and behavioral interventions for the client exhibiting aggression, hostility, and violence. (p. 601–602)

_____

_____

_____

8. List legal and ethical issues related to violence. (p. 606)

_____

_____

_____

Case Study

Suggested answers for Case Studies are provided in the Answers section at the back of this Study Guide.

Scenario:
A recent psychiatric admission to a locked unit demands to have his cigarettes. Per hospital policy, no smoking is allowed in the building or on the grounds. As his request is denied, the client raises his voice, slams his fist into the wall, and yells, "I better get a smoke or you will pay!"

1. What should be the nurse's first verbal response?

_____

_____

_____

_____

2. How can other staff be of assistance at this time?

_____

_____

_____

_____

_____

3. What causative factors may have contributed to this client's outburst?

_____

_____

_____

_____

_____

4. What interventions may the nurse use in this situation?

_____

_____

_____

_____

_____

Self-Assessment Questions

Answers and rationales for Self-Assessment Questions are provided in the Answers section at the back of this Study Guide.

1. Which of the following examples is a form of acting out?
    a.   Putting a fist through a window
    b.   Being involved in the school play
    c.   Joining an exercise class
    d.   Playing a video role-playing game

2. A client is out of control, and the nurse has determined that he is a danger to others. Which of the following statements by the nurse is most therapeutic in this situation?
    a.   "Sir, you have two choices. You can calm down or we will help you to calm down."
    b.   "Sir, calm down or I will give you a shot."
    c.   "Sir, we can handle any behavior you wish to show us."
    d.   "Sir, don't you dare hurt anyone."

3. Which documentation in a client's chart provides a nurse with the greatest legal protection?
    a.   "Client placed in seclusion per policy."
    b.   "Client was given choice to calm down or be helped to calm down. Client chose to be helped to the quiet room."
    c.   "Client was administered a sedative with assistance."
    d.   "After client threatened his roommate, the client was forced to the floor."

4. A mental health assistant on an adolescent inpatient psychiatric unit makes the following comment: "That kid is just plain bad. His parents just didn't discipline him enough." The nurse's best response is:

    a. "You are probably right. Adolescents who end up here should have had stronger discipline as they were growing up."

    b. "I agree. Some kids are just out of control for no reason."

    c. "Actually, studies have found that behavior like his is highly heritable."

    d. "His parents should have had classes on discipline long ago."

5. Three of the following strategies are priorities for a safe work environment. Which strategy is least effective?

    a. Providing emergency department and psychiatric staff with wireless panic buttons

    b. Implementing a "code" protocol to assist staff with violent situations

    c. Offering self-defense classes after work

    d. Installing good lighting in the hallways and parking lots

6. Which of the following is a risk factor for violence?

    a. Growing up in a large family

    b. Working in a large office with several employees

    c. Working in an area with visible security officers

    d. Having open access to the work building

7. Which of the following statements by a client indicates a characteristic associated with violence?

    a. "It's not my fault I got fired again. It was that stupid supervisor."

    b. "I get so angry when I forget to balance my checkbook."

    c. "Even though I don't like my job, it pays the bills."

    d. "I may not be the most outgoing guy, but at least I stand up for myself."

8. A client comes up to the nurses' station and yells, "Where are my pills? I asked for them an hour ago. If I don't get them soon, someone is going to pay!" Which statement by the nurse would help de-escalate the situation?

    a. "I can understand you are upset, how can I help you?"

    b. "I'll get your meds as soon as you go to your room."

    c. "I won't help you because you are yelling."

    d. "I can't help you when you are yelling."

CHAPTER 21

The Client with a Substance-Related Disorder

This chapter provides a comprehensive account of some of the causes of substance abuse and the theories surrounding these disorders. The role of the nurse in caring for individuals with a substance-related disorder is addressed, including the importance of maintaining a caring attitude when working with clients who abuse substances.

Reading Assignment

Prior to beginning this assignment, please read Chapter 21, "The Client with a Substance-Related Disorder."

Activities

Using the content in the text, answer the following questions as clearly as you can and in your own words. Give examples, if appropriate, to help clarify the information in your answer.

1. Compare and contrast the *DSM-IV-TR* criteria for substance abuse and substance dependence. (Table 21–1, pp. 621–622)

   _____

   _____

   _____

   _____

   _____

   _____

2. Compare and contrast the *DSM-IV-TR* criteria for substance intoxication and substance withdrawal. (Table 21–1, pp. 621–622)

   _____

   _____

   _____

3. Name and explain the theories surrounding substance-related disorders. (pp. 628–631)

a. _____
_____
_____

b. _____
_____
_____
_____

c. _____
_____
_____
_____

d. _____
_____
_____
_____

e. _____
_____
_____
_____

f. _____
_____
_____
_____

g. _____
_____
_____
_____

h. _____
_____
_____
_____

i. _____
_____
_____

4. Complete the following table, including blood alcohol levels (concentrations) and related effects. (Table 21–3, p. 633)

Blood Alcohol Level (BAL) and Effects

BAL	Number of Drinks		Effects
	Male	Female	

5. What are some of the medical consequences of alcoholism? (Table 21–4, p. 633)

6. What are the main areas of assessment on the CIWA tool? (Table 21–5, pp. 635–636)

a.

b.

c.

d.

e.

f.

g.

7. Summarize the various models of treatment for individuals who abuse substances. (p. 647)

a.

b.

c.

d.

e.

f.

g.

8. Assessment of individuals with substance-related disorders includes: (p. 651)

   a. _____

   b. _____

   c. _____

   d. _____

   e. _____

   f. _____

   g. _____

   h. _____

9. What are the symptoms of overdose for the following substances? (Table 21–9, pp. 653–654)

   a. Alcohol _____

   _____

   _____

   b. Opiates _____

   _____

   _____

   c. Sedative-hypnotics _____

   _____

   _____

   d. Stimulants _____

   _____

   _____

   e. Cannabis _____

   _____

   _____

   f. Inhalants _____

   _____

   _____

   g. Hallucinogens _____

   _____

   _____

   h. Caffeine _____

   _____

   _____

   i. Nicotine_____

   _____

   _____

10. What are the manifestations of withdrawal syndrome for the following substances?
     (Table 21–9, pp. 653–654)

     a. Alcohol _____

     _____

     _____

     b. Opiates _____

     _____

     _____

     c. Sedative-hypnotics _____

     _____

     _____

     d. Stimulants _____

     _____

     _____

     e. Cannabis _____

     _____

     _____

     f. Inhalants _____

     _____

     _____

     g. Hallucinogens _____

     _____

     _____

     h. Caffeine _____

     _____

     _____

     i. Nicotine _____

     _____

     _____

11. Describe *DSM-IV-TR* and the older adult with alcohol problems. (Table 21–8, p. 657)

     _____

     _____

     _____

     _____

     _____

     _____

     _____

     _____

_____

_____

Case Study

Suggested answers for Case Studies are provided in the Answers section at the back of this Study Guide.

Scenario:
A middle-aged female drinks between 8 and 12 cans of beer per day. Her first drink each day is upon awakening. She has been drinking alcohol on a regular basis since high school. Although she has had numerous jobs, she is either fired or quits within a month or two of being hired. She has lived off and on with many boyfriends and occasionally comes home to her parents and stays for several weeks. She has been known to pawn items from her parents' home to support her drinking habit.

1. What physical assessments should be made?

_____

_____

_____

2. What family dynamics should be explored?

_____

_____

_____

3. Describe the disease concept associated with alcoholism.

_____

_____

_____

4. Describe the effects of addiction to alcohol on the family.

_____

_____

_____

Self-Assessment Questions

Answers and rationales for Self-Assessment Questions are provided in the Answers section at the back of this Study Guide.

1. A client with a substance abuse disorder makes the comment, "Lately, I have had to get more and more of my drug just to get the effect I used to get." The nurse analyzes this as an example of:
   a. Addiction
   b. Dependence
   c. Tolerance
   d. Withdrawal

2. A client has had surgery and is recovering in the intensive care unit 72 hours after he was first admitted. The client exhibits tremors, jumps in a jerky manner when anyone enters the room, has a heart rate of 132, has a 101° fever, and complains of bugs in his room. An immediate assessment question that should be asked by the nurse is:

   a. "When was your last drink?"

   b. "Does schizophrenia run in your family?"

   c. "What is your pain level on a scale of 1 to 10?"

   d. "Have you been around anyone with the stomach flu?"

3. A client has had surgery and is recovering in the intensive care unit 72 hours after he was first admitted. The client exhibits tremors, jumps in a jerky manner when anyone enters the room, has a heart rate of 132, has several loose stools, and complains of bugs in his room. The nurse should take the following action:

   a. Document the signs and symptoms and call them to the attention of the surgeon when he makes rounds

   b. Leave a message for the health care provider to consider ordering an antipsychotic

   c. Notify the doctor immediately of suspected alcohol withdrawal and ask for orders

   d. Refer the client for an alcohol evaluation

4. A client has had surgery and is recovering in the intensive care unit 72 hours after he was first admitted. The client exhibits tremors, jumps in a jerky manner when anyone enters the room, has a heart rate of 132, has several loose stools, and complains of bugs in his room. After calling the doctor, the nurse enters the room and the client begins to have a seizure. The nurse again calls the physician to update the client's condition. The nurse should anticipate which initial action by the physician?

   a. Administer parental thiamine

   b. Administer parental anxiolytic medication, such as chlordiazepoxide (Librium) or lorazepam (Ativan)

   c. Order restraints

   d. Transfer to psychiatric unit

5. A client has had surgery and is recovering in the intensive care unit 72 hours after he was first admitted. The client exhibits tremors, jumps in a jerky manner when anyone enters the room, has a heart rate of 132, has several loose stools, and complains of bugs in his room. After calling the doctor, the nurse enters the room and the client begins to seizure. What is the priority nursing diagnosis?

   a. Risk for injury

   b. Ineffective denial

   c. Ineffective coping

   d. Imbalanced nutrition

6. Three of the following questions are expected when completing a Clinical Institute Withdrawal Assessment-Alcohol Tool. Which question would not be included in the assessment?

   a. "Does the color of the room appear different to you?"

   b. "Do you have itchy skin?"

   c. "Do you feel sick to your stomach?"

   d. "Do you have pain in the area of your liver?"

7. Following major surgery, a client denies pain and refuses all analgesics. The nurse observes that the client lies still in bed, is diaphoretic, moans, and is guarded. When challenged about whether he is feeling acute pain, the client admits, "I am in a lot of pain, but I don't want to take anything so I won't get addicted." The best response by the nurse is:
   a. "It is true that if you take narcotics and are already having trouble with a drug dependency, the narcotics will make you worse."
   b. "The likelihood of causing you to become drug dependent is practically nonexistent."
   c. "That is why we wait until your pain is high before we give the next dose."
   d. "There are worse things than feeling pain."

8. A client at the community mental health clinic complains of insomnia. He has trouble falling asleep and staying asleep. Which of the following data should be explored further by the advanced-practice psychiatric nurse?
   a. "I run at least a mile every day after work about 5 p.m."
   b. "I go to bed anywhere between 11 p.m. and midnight every night."
   c. "I drink a cola every morning when I wake up and usually four or five more each day."
   d. "On the weekend, I try to catch a nap."

9. Which comment by a client with alcoholism indicates he has accepted the first of the 12 steps of Alcoholics Anonymous?
   a. "Alcohol is stronger than I am."
   b. "I have to make apologies to my family and try to make things right again."
   c. "I have done a lot of things wrong in my life."
   d. "I've made this list of things, both good and bad, about myself."

10. Which statement by the client being discharged from an alcohol treatment center would indicate that further teaching is necessary?
    a. "I can have a glass of wine on a special occasion."
    b. "I will have to talk with my sponsor every day or more often."
    c. "I will need to go to Alcoholics Anonymous regularly, even when I don't think I need it."
    d. "I don't have to adopt all the 12 steps, but I will keep an open mind about them."

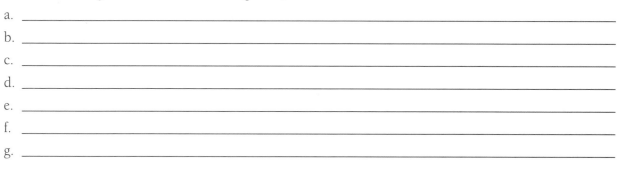

CHAPTER 22

The Client with an Eating Disorder

This chapter looks at some of the causes of eating disorders and the treatment modalities related to these disorders. The nurse is exposed to various theories surrounding these disorders and means of implementing care through use of the nursing process approach.

Reading Assignment

Prior to beginning this assignment, please read Chapter 22, "The Client with an Eating Disorder."

Activities

Using the content in the text, answer the following questions as clearly as you can and in your own words. Give examples, if appropriate, to help clarify the information in your answer.

1. What are the major features of anorexia? (p. 675)

   a. _____

   b. _____

   c. _____

   d. _____

   e. _____

   f. _____

   g. _____

2. Identify the physiological findings in eating disorders. (Table 22–1, p. 677)

Physiological Findings in Eating Disorders

Category	Abnormal Finding(s)

3. Compare and contrast the *DSM-IV-TR* criteria for bulimia nervosa and anorexia nervosa. (pp. 676, 678)

    • _____

    • _____

    • _____

    • _____

4. Compare and contrast the *DSM-IV-TR* criteria for binge eating disorder, pica, and rumination. (p. 678)

    • _____

    • _____

    • _____

    • _____

    • _____

5. List some of the co-occurring conditions that occur with eating disorders. (pp. 675–677)

    a. _____

    b. _____

    c. _____

    d. _____

    e. _____

6. Identify the theories and causative factors related to eating disorders. (pp. 681–683)

    • _____

    • _____

    • _____

    • _____

    • _____

7. Explain the treatment modalities for eating disorders. (pp. 685–689)

    a. _____

    b. _____

    c. _____

    d. _____

    e. _____

8. Relate laboratory tests for clients with eating disorders. (p. 688)

    a. _____

    b. _____

    c. _____

    d. _____

    e. _____

    f. _____

    g. _____

    h. _____

    i. _____

    j. _____

9. Identify the symptoms that are present in a client with an eating disorder. (Table 22–6, p. 688)

Physiological Assessment in Eating Disorders

	Anorexia	Bulimia
Gastrointestinal		
Cardiovascular		
Endocrine		
Pulmonary		
Dermatological		
Renal		

10. Calculate your own BMI. (p. 671)

    _____

    _____

    _____

    _____

11. Nursing interventions used with a client with anorexia or bulimia are: (pp. 694–695)

    a. _____

    b. _____

    c. _____

    d. _____

    e. _____

f. _____

g. _____

h. _____

12. Interventions for management of a client with anorexia nervosa include: (pp. 685–687)

    a. _____

    b. _____

    c. _____

    d. _____

    e. _____

    f. _____

    g. _____

    h. _____

    i. _____

    j. _____

13. Interventions for management of a client with bulimia nervosa include: (pp. 685–687)

    a. _____

    b. _____

    c. _____

    d. _____

    e. _____

    f. _____

    g. _____

    h. _____

    i. _____

    j. _____

Case Study

Suggested answers for Case Studies are provided in the Answers section at the back of this Study Guide.

Scenario:
A 20-year-old female is diagnosed with anorexia nervosa. As a teenager, she was never overweight but was never thin. She was active in sports, and a coach commented that she would perform better if she lost a few pounds. She lost over 40 pounds, and she weighed 85 pounds and was 5 feet 2 inches when she was first diagnosed. Her parents, both with professional careers, put her in treatment at the recommendation of the physician. For the last 3 years, the client has struggled to gain weight and currently weighs 89 pounds.

1. What lab values are important to monitor for this client?

    _____

    _____

    _____

2. What family dynamics are important to consider?

_____

_____

_____

3. What treatment modalities could be used for this client?

_____

_____

_____

Self-Assessment Questions

Answers and rationales for Self-Assessment Questions are provided in the Answers section at the back of this Study Guide.

1. Which of the following health care professionals may be the first to suspect bulimia nervosa?

   a.   Dentist

   b.   Nurse

   c.   Physician

   d.   Occupational therapist

2. A female who is 5 feet 2 inches tall and weighs 82 pounds is hospitalized for anorexia nervosa. During recreational therapy, the client gets ready to go swimming. When the client sees herself in the mirror, she states, "Oh my, I am so fat." The nurse observes a skeletal figure with all ribs evident and bony prominences pronounced. The nurse's best assessment of the client's comment is:

   a.   The client is seeking attention.

   b.   The client is hallucinating.

   c.   The client is experiencing an illusion.

   d.   The client has body image disturbance.

3. The school nurse is conducting routine health screens. One 14-year-old female is observed wearing a large sweater over a bulky sweatshirt. Her hair is dry and unmanageable, with patches of scalp showing. Her shoes are tight fitting and her arms have fine hair from wrist to elbow. The nurse understands that these symptoms are consistent with which of the following disorders?

   a.   Pica

   b.   Bulimia

   c.   Dehydration

   d.   Anorexia nervosa

4. A mother of a teenager was heard saying, "I just couldn't be prouder of my girl. Look at how slim and trim she is, even though she is a big eater. Other than the fact that she disappears right after every meal for about 20 minutes, she gives me no problems." These comments are consistent with which eating disorders?

    a. Binge eating disorder

    b. Anorexia nervosa

    c. Pica

    d. Bulimia nervosa

5. An adolescent is being seen in the community mental health clinic for pica. Her mother has accompanied her to the clinic. Which statement by the mother indicates that further teaching is necessary?

    a. "I'll need to make sure she has more zinc and iron in her diet."

    b. "Pica is eating nonnutritive substances."

    c. "I will have to watch her after meals to make sure she isn't vomiting."

    d. "There is a concern for an intestinal obstruction."

6. Which of the following persons is among the population with the most risk for developing an eating disorder?

    a. Football player

    b. Balance beam gymnast

    c. Health professional

    d. Singer

7. Which of the following physical assessments are found on examination of a client with anorexia nervosa? Select all that apply.

    a. Constipation

    b. Alopecia

    c. Tachycardia

    d. Hypertension

    e. Amenorrhea

    f. Oily skin

    g. Decreased BUN

    h. Electrocardiographic (EEG) abnormalities

8. Using the following formula, calculate the body mass index of a client who is 5 feet 2 inches tall and weighs 81 pounds.

    $$\frac{\text{Weight (kg)}}{\text{Height (m)}^2}$$

    _____

9. A client has gone from 115 pounds to 75 pounds within the last 6 months. The client continues to diet and exercise. Her typical food is five flakes of cereal for breakfast, one apple slice for lunch, and one-fourth of one slice of cheese for an evening meal. She drinks eight glasses of water each day. What is the primary nursing diagnosis for this client?

   a. Imbalanced nutrition: less than body requirements

   b. Deficient fluid volume

   c. Ineffective coping

   d. Disturbed body image

10. A client has gone from 115 pounds to 75 pounds within the last 6 months. The client continues to diet and exercise. Her typical food is five flakes of cereal for breakfast, one apple slice for lunch, and one-fourth of one slice of cheese for an evening meal. She drinks eight glasses of water each day. What is the priority nursing intervention for this client?

   a. Intake of nutrition either by the client or through a nasogastric tube

   b. Calculate the caloric intake

   c. Develop a behavior modification program

   d. Document intake and output

—NOTES—

CHAPTER 23

The Client with a Sleep Disorder

The range of sleep disorders is discussed in this chapter, including the evidence of sleep disorders across the life span. Various treatment modalities are presented, with emphasis on the importance of maintaining healthy routines to encourage good sleep habits.

Reading Assignment

Prior to beginning this assignment, please read Chapter 23, "The Client with a Sleep Disorder."

Activities

Using the content in the text, answer the following questions as clearly as you can and in your own words. Give examples, if appropriate, to help clarify the information in your answer.

1. Relate the stages of sleep to the physiological changes in the body. (Table 23–1, p. 704)

Non–Rapid Eye Movement Sleep Stages

Stage	Physiological Process

2. Compare and contrast the medical conditions and psychiatric conditions that cause insomnia. (Table 23–2, p. 707)

_____   _____

_____   _____

_____   _____

_____   _____

_____   _____

_____   _____

_____   _____

_____   _____

_____   _____

3. List the medications that cause insomnia. (Table 23–2, p. 707)

_____   _____

_____   _____

_____   _____

_____   _____

_____   _____

4. Describe how sleep disorders are manifested across the life span. (pp. 710–712)

Developmental Perspectives on Sleep Disorders

Stages of Life	Sleep Disturbance(s)
Infancy and childhood	
Adolescence	
Adulthood	
Older adulthood	

In the following tables, fill in the correct information about pharmacologic agents to treat insomnia and specific medical conditions.

5. Indicate the side effects and specific nursing implications for benzodiazepines. (Table 23–3, p. 713)

Benzodiazepines	Side Effects	Nursing Implications

6. Indicate the side effects and specific nursing implications for nonbenzodiazepines. (Table 23–3, p. 713)

Nonbenzodiazepines	Side Effects	Nursing Implications

7. Indicate the side effects and specific nursing implications for tricyclic antidepressants. (Table 23–3, p. 713)

Antidepressants (Tricyclic)	Side Effects	Nursing Implications

8. Indicate the side effects and specific nursing implications for novel antidepressants. (Table 23–3, p. 713)

Antidepressants	Side Effects	Nursing Implications

9. Indicate the side effects and specific nursing implications for anticonvulsants. (Table 23–3, p. 714)

Anticonvulsants	Side Effects	Nursing Implications

10. Identify some of the behaviors that you have observed in clients you have worked with in clinical experiences that should be maintained in order to promote good sleep hygiene. (Table 23–4, p. 715)

a. _____
b. _____
c. _____
d. _____
e. _____
f. _____
g. _____
h. _____
i. _____
j. _____
k. _____
l. _____
m. _____
n. _____
o. _____
p. _____

11. Identify some of the nursing diagnoses that are appropriate for use with clients who have sleep disorders. (p. 716)

a. _____
b. _____
c. _____
d. _____
e. _____
f. _____

12. List specific goals that may be used for clients with a sleep disorder. (p. 717)

a. _____

b. _____

c. _____

d. _____

e. _____

Case Study

Suggested answers for Case Studies are provided in the Answers section at the back of this Study Guide.

Scenario:
A college-aged student is failing classes. He reports a great deal of difficulty waking up to go to class. He sleeps most of the day and finds he has the most energy after 6 p.m. each day. Although he sets several alarms to awaken in time to go to class, he sleeps through the alarms.

1. What should be included in the assessment of this client?

_____

_____

_____

2. What therapies might be beneficial to this client?

_____

_____

_____

3. What nursing diagnosis is consistent with the client's behavior?

_____

_____

_____

Self-Assessment Questions

Answers and rationales for Self-Assessment Questions are provided in the Answers section at the back of this Study Guide.

1. In which non–rapid eye movement stage of sleep is growth hormone released?
   a. Stage I
   b. Stage II
   c. Stage II
   d. Stage IV

2. A peer complains that it is increasingly more difficult to fall asleep at night. The peer describes lying in bed and her mind continuing to race. Which statement by the peer indicates a need to challenge the peer's activity?

    a. "I have a lot of energy, so I usually jog when I get home from work at 5 p.m."

    b. "I love my hot chocolate while I curl up and watch the 10 p.m. news."

    c. "I have taken a multivitamin every morning for years."

    d. "I take 81 milligrams of aspirin every other day to prevent heart disease."

3. Which of the statements by the client with a sleep disorder indicates that further teaching is necessary?

    a. "If I can't fall asleep at night, I should just lie there and force myself to relax anyway."

    b. "I should plan to go to bed and get up on a regular schedule every day."

    c. "I should turn the TV off a couple of hours before going to bed."

    d. "I should take my diuretic in the morning instead of at night."

4. A client at the community mental health clinic states that his wife has found him talking in the garage at 2 a.m., but he has no recollection of how he got to the garage. This behavior is an example of:

    a. Sleep apnea

    b. Nightmare disorder

    c. Hypersomnia

    d. Sleepwalking

5. During the admission to a surgical floor, the nurse conducts an assessment. The client complains of fatigue and difficulty sleeping. An important question to ask to further clarify the client's sleep disturbance is:

    a. "How would you characterize your stress at work?"

    b. "Tell me about your routine sleep habits."

    c. "How did you sleep when you were a child?"

    d. "Do your family members have trouble sleeping?"

6. A client falls asleep without difficulty but awakens very early and is unable to fall back asleep. Which mental illness is most closely associated with this sleep disturbance?

    a. Bipolar disorder

    b. Major depressive disorder

    c. Cyclothymia

    d. Schizophrenia

7. Which of the following bedtime activities can promote sleep?

    a. Eating a bowl of cereal

    b. Drinking hot chocolate

    c. Drinking a glass of wine

    d. Doing exercise

—NOTES—

CHAPTER 24

The Client with a Sexual Disorder

For the nurse, sexual disorders may be difficult to understand. This chapter addresses the causes of these disorders and looks at the psychosocial and neurobiological factors that provide the basis for care to these clients.

Reading Assignment

Prior to beginning this assignment, please read Chapter 24, "The Client with a Sexual Disorder."

Activities

Using the content in the text, answer the following questions as clearly as you can and in your own words. Give examples, if appropriate, to help clarify the information in your answer.

1. Relate the various theories and perspectives to sexuality. (pp. 732–733)

   Psychoanalytic theory _____

   _____

   _____

   Behavioral theory _____

   _____

   _____

   Social learning theory _____

   _____

   _____

   Self-actualization theories _____

   _____

   _____

Sociological theories _____

_____

_____

2. Compare and contrast the specific sexual and gender disorders as identified in the *DSM-IV-TR*. (Table 24–2, p. 740)

a. _____

b. _____

c. _____

d. _____

e. _____

f. _____

g. _____

h. _____

i. _____

3. List the various medical conditions that contribute to sexual dysfunction. (Table 24–3, p. 742)

Medical Conditions That Affect Sexual Function

Areas Affected	Effects

4. List the classifications and types of drugs that affect sexual function. (Table 24–4, p. 743)

Drugs That Affect Sexual Function

Classification	Types of Drugs

Case Study

Suggested answers for Case Studies are provided in the Answers section at the back of this Study Guide.

Scenario:
The husband of a depressed client states that his wife has lost all interest in sexual activity since she has been diagnosed. Although he is supportive of his wife during her illness, he struggles with the lack of intimacy in his marriage. He is requesting couples' counseling from the community mental health clinic.

1. What assessment activities should be included during the initial interview?

_____

_____

_____

2. What psychosocial cause might be considered in this situation?

_____

_____

_____

3. What neurobiological factor is important in this situation?

_____

_____

_____

4. Describe the role of the advanced-practice psychiatric nurse in working with this couple.

_____

_____

_____

Self-Assessment Questions

Answers and rationales for Self-Assessment Questions are provided in the Answers section at the back of this Study Guide.

1. Following bypass surgery, a middle-aged man asks the nurse, "Since sex is a big part of my marriage, how will I give that up now that I have this heart problem?" The nurse's most appropriate response is:
    a. "I realize that your surgery has been scary for you, but it doesn't mean your sex life is over."
    b. "There are many ways you can show each other your love other than through sex."
    c. "If you pace yourself, you should be able to enjoy sex once in awhile."
    d. "There are medications that can diminish one's desire."

2. A young mother asks the clinic pediatric nurse how she should approach sex education with her teenage daughter. The best response by the nurse is:
    a. "Your daughter will ask you when she is ready to learn about the subject."
    b. "Your daughter's school will have a health class on it very soon."
    c. "It is often a mistake to wait for children to ask for information."
    d. "Take these brochures and leave them in an area in the house where she will find them."

3. A 24-year-old male has abruptly quit taking escitalopram (Lexapro) for his depression. The community mental health nurse asks him to explain his decision. He states, "Because I was unable to come to climax with my partner. It wasn't worth it." The nurse's best response is:

    a.   "There are serious consequences of quitting your medication."

    b.   "I understand the side effect is undesirable, but so is the depression you have been experiencing."

    c.   "Both your mental health and your intimate relationship are important to you."

    d.   "You did the right thing by stopping the medication."

4. A nursing home resident has been married for 51 years. The resident's husband visits daily. The client is alert and oriented to time, place, and person but has had a cerebral vascular accident that requires long-term care for her paralysis. Several times a month, the husband goes to his wife's single room and shuts the door with a "Do Not Disturb" sign posted to the door. The nursing assistant asks the charge nurse if he can legally do that. The nurse's best response is:

    a.   "As long as we check on them every few minutes, it is OK to have the door shut for a short time."

    b.   "We'll need to keep the door open at all times so we can monitor their activity."

    c.   "They have a right to privacy for several hours if they would like."

    d.   "We'll have to get a doctor's order before we can allow it."

5. A graduate student is under pressure to finish his thesis. To alleviate the stresses of his program of study, he uses marijuana. At first he smoked occasionally on the weekends. Now he states he uses "weed" at least three or four times a week. He has begun fighting with his partner over small things. He states he has had several incidences of impotence. The nurse attributes the student's impotence problems to:

    a.   Marijuana use

    b.   Stress of school

    c.   Relationship stressors

    d.   Age

6. During a routine visit with her primary care provider, a client reports that her mental health provider ordered venlafaxine XR and later added bupropion to her medication regimen. She also reports sexual side effects from the venlafaxine. She asks the nurse, "Why do I need to take two antidepressants? Am I that sick that I need to take two pills?" The most appropriate response by the nurse is:

    a.   "Sometimes bupropion is ordered to reduce the sexual side effects of venlafaxine."

    b.   "Continue taking the venlafaxine and bupropion as ordered."

    c.   "Stop taking the bupropion until your provider explains reasons for this medication."

    d.   "Wait until your next appointment and ask your mental health provider why bupropion was added."

7. A co-worker makes a derogatory remark about the sexual orientation of a gay patient. When challenged on her comment, she responds, "Well, the American Psychiatric Association lists homosexuality as a mental disorder worthy of diagnosis. That must mean it should be treated like a disease." The most appropriate response is:

    a.   "It is true that the APA did have homosexuality as a mental disorder, but it is no longer categorized as a mental disorder."

    b.   "It is listed as a mental disorder because homosexuals live a stressful life due to society's judgmental attitude about it."

    c.   "Treatment for homosexuality is often unsuccessful."

    d.   "The APA has never, nor will it ever, list homosexuality as a mental disorder needing treatment."

CHAPTER 25

The Client Who Survives Violence

Violence crosses the entire life span. For that reason it is important for all nurses to be adequately prepared to correctly assess victims of violence and implement care as needed. This chapter addresses violence from every aspect, from some of the causative factors of abuse to the role of the nurse in each phase of care through the nursing process.

Reading Assignment

Prior to beginning this assignment, please read Chapter 25, "The Client Who Survives Violence."

Activities

Using the content in the text, answer the following questions as clearly as you can and in your own words. Give examples, if appropriate, to help clarify the information in your answer.

1. List the signs and symptoms of shaken baby syndrome. (Table 25–2, p. 758)

   a. _____

   b. _____

   c. _____

   d. _____

   e. _____

   f. _____

   g. _____

   h. _____

   i. _____

2. Identify the types of sexual abuse behaviors. (Table 25–4, p. 760)

   - _____
   - _____
   - _____
   - _____
   - _____
   - _____
   - _____
   - _____

3. Identify the myths and corresponding facts about intimate partner violence. (p. 765)

Myths about Intimate Partner Violence

Myth	Fact

4. Identify the principles as delineated by Warshaw that should be followed in working with survivors of intimate partner violence. (p. 765)

   a. _____

   b. _____

   c. _____

   d. _____

   e. _____

5. Identify some of the causative factors of abuse. Briefly explain these theories as they relate to abuse. (pp. 768–771)

Causative Factors of Abuse

Theory	Explanation

6. Identify the risk factors (psychosocial factors) for child abuse. (p. 773)

    • _____

    • _____

    • _____

    • _____

    • _____

7. List the eight propositions that, according to Straus, illustrate how general systems theory relates to family violence. (p. 770)

    a. _____

    _____

    b. _____

    _____

    c. _____

    _____

    d. _____

    _____

    e. _____

    _____

    f. _____

    _____

    g. _____

    _____

    h. _____

    _____

8. What are some of the immediate effects of abuse on the child and adolescent? (Table 25–5, p. 761)

Immediate Effects of Abuse on the Child and Adolescent

Area to Be Assessed	Effects

9. Abuse affects the family of the victim as well. List the acute and chronic effects of abuse on the family. (Table 25–6, p. 772)

Effects of Abuse on the Family

Acute	Chronic

10. Identify some of the issues that are addressed in individual therapy involving clients who survive violence. (p. 774)

a. _____

b. _____

c. _____

d. _____

e. _____

f. _____

g. _____

h. _____

i. _____

j. _____

11. Identify some of the issues that may be discussed in family therapy involving clients who survive violence. (pp. 774–775)

a. _____

b. _____

c. _____

d. _____

e. _____

f. _____

g. _____

h. _____

i. _____

j. _____

12. Various therapies may be used to assist children in dealing with violence. These interventions include: (p. 776)

a. _____

b. _____

c. _____

d. _____

e. _____

f. _____

g. _____

Case Study

Suggested answers for Case Studies are provided in the Answers section at the back of this Study Guide.

Scenario:
An adolescent girl is returned to her family after having been abducted at gunpoint from a shopping mall and taken out of state. Her abductor molested her during the 2 weeks she was missing. She was able to escape by running away while the abductor slept.

1. What is the priority consideration in reintegrating the teenager back into the family?

_____

_____

_____

_____

_____

2. What nursing interventions should the advanced-practice psychiatric nurse use when working with the family?

_____

_____

_____

_____

_____

Self-Assessment Questions

Answers and rationales for Self-Assessment Questions are provided in the Answers section at the back of this Study Guide.

1. A family member brings a 7-year-old girl into the emergency department. The complaint is a head injury related to "falling off my bicycle." During the examination, numerous bruises are noted on the child's thin frame in various stages of healing. The girl is vague in answering how she got the older bruises. The nurse needs to collect further data for suspected:

a. Child abuse

b. Knowledge deficit pertaining to child safety

c. Normal behavior for a 7-year-old

d. Suicidal gestures

2. An elderly woman is being seen for a routine annual physical by the advanced-practice psychiatric nurse. Observations note that the woman has lost 21 pounds since her last visit a year earlier. Her clothes are loose, and the woman has a difficult time keeping her slacks from falling off her hips. Her daughter, with whom the woman lives, answers all questions for her mother. What should be the nurse practitioner's initial action?

   a.   Refer the family to a nutritionist

   b.   Request the daughter leave the examination room

   c.   Initiate teaching about nutritional supplements

   d.   Request an evaluation by the social worker to begin placement out of the daughter's home

3. An elderly woman is being seen for a routine annual physical by the advanced-practice psychiatric nurse. Observations note that the woman has lost 21 pounds since her last visit a year earlier. Her clothes are loose and the woman has a difficult time keeping her slacks from falling off her hips. Her daughter, with whom the woman lives, answers all questions for her mother. Neglect is suspected. The best course of action is:

   a.   Notify adult protective services

   b.   Teach the daughter to feed her mother high-calorie foods

   c.   Initiate the board of mental health proceedings

   d.   Refer the daughter for individual psychotherapy

4. An elderly woman is being seen for a routine annual physical by the advanced-practice psychiatric nurse. Observations note that the woman has lost 21 pounds since her last visit a year earlier. Her clothes are loose and the woman has a difficult time keeping her slacks from falling off her hips. Her daughter, with whom the woman lives, answers all questions for her mother. When the nurse practitioner asks the daughter how things are going at home, the daughter answers, "I am exhausted. I work two jobs and have three children still at home." Which response by the nurse would indicate the nurse has an understanding of the caregiver's stress?

   a.   "You need to hire some help."

   b.   "Here are some brochures on caring for parents."

   c.   "It can be very demanding caring for loved ones."

   d.   "Have you thought about putting her in a nursing home?"

5. A female college student goes to the campus health center to see the nurse practitioner for a possible broken finger and bruises. She admits that her boyfriend had a few too many drinks the night before and got "rough with me." The nurse practitioner's most appropriate response is:

   a.   "You need to break it off with your boyfriend for your own sake."

   b.   "You should press charges."

   c.   "Here are some resources on campus to help you work this all out."

   d.   "Your safety is important to me. Let's talk about some things you might want to consider."

6. Which of the following symptoms are consistent with shaken baby syndrome? List all that apply.
   a. Limp arms and legs
   b. Lusty, loud cry when laid on the examination table
   c. Puffy, protruding fontanels
   d. Constricted pupils
   e. Difficulty arousing from sleep
   f. Tachycardia
   g. Elevated temperature

7. A young mother and her two children have just arrived at the emergency shelter for battered women. During the support group, the mother states, "Finally I am safe. It took a lot to up and leave. I will never hear from him again." The community mental health nurse who is leading the group should include which of the following concepts in her response:
   a. Women who leave their batterers are still in danger of harm.
   b. The location of the shelter is protected, and her batterer will not be able to find her or the children.
   c. The legal system will provide her ample protection.
   d. Spousal abuse is not connected to child abuse, so her children are safe.

8. A teenage girl is admitted to the psychiatric adolescent unit for a suicide attempt. She overdosed on her mother's medication. Her arms have numerous scars and fresh wounds. When questioned about the wounds to her arms, she admits cutting herself, saying, "When I see the blood, I know I am still alive." Her history indicates that she has not been to school for 2 weeks and she has been living at 'friends' homes instead of going home at night. The nurse should collect further data regarding which of the following?
   a. Pregnancy
   b. Sexual abuse by someone in the home
   c. Bulimia nervosa
   d. Conduct disorder

9. Which comment about intimate partner violence by a student indicates that further teaching is necessary?
   a. "Intimate partner violence has to have some sort of physical evidence to be diagnosed."
   b. "Both men and women can be involved in causing intimate partner violence."
   c. "Intimate partner violence involves guns most of the time."
   d. "Men are raped as a result of intimate partner violence."

10. During the course of an examination, a female client states, "My boyfriend won't let me get my hair cut unless I check with him first. And then he has to approve how it will be cut too." The nurses analyzes this comment as:
    a. A patriarchal relationship
    b. Inconsequential
    c. Potential physical abuse
    d. Intimate partner violence

—NOTES—

UNIT 3

Therapeutic Interventions

Chapter 26   Individual Psychotherapy

Chapter 27   Group Therapy

Chapter 28   Familial Systems and Family Therapy

Chapter 29   Psychopharmacologic Therapy

Chapter 30   Electroconvulsive, Other Biological (Somatic), and Complementary Therapies

Chapter 31   Crisis Intervention Management: The Role of Adaptation

Chapter 32   Milieu Therapy/Hospital-Based Care

Chapter 33   Home- and Community-Based Care

Chapter 34   Psychosocial Care in Medical-Surgical Settings

CHAPTER 26

Individual Psychotherapy

This chapter gives the basic background for understanding the theories and concepts of individual psychotherapy. The role of the nurse is emphasized, with identification of specific interventions to be provided by generalists and advanced-practice psychiatric nurses.

Reading Assignment

Prior to beginning this assignment, please read Chapter 26, "Individual Psychotherapy."

Activities

Using the content in the text, answer the following questions as clearly as you can and in your own words. Give examples, if appropriate, to help clarify the information in your answer.

1. Identify the types of psychotherapy, and stage goals and other features of each. (Table 26–1, p. 792)

Psychotherapies: Theoretical Approaches

Type	Goal	Specific Illness/Indication	Duration	Techniques

2. Explain the major treatment techniques of psychoanalytical psychotherapy. (p. 792–793)

_____

_____

_____

_____

_____

3. Discuss the technique of brief psychotherapy and the goals related to this procedure. (p. 794)

_____

_____

_____

_____

_____

4. Discuss the technique of interpersonal psychotherapy and the goals related to this procedure. (p. 794)

_____

_____

_____

_____

_____

5. Discuss the technique of stress-reducing therapy and the goals related to this procedure. (p. 794)

_____

_____

_____

_____

_____

6. Discuss the technique of behavioral therapy and the goals related to this procedure. (pp. 794–795)

_____

_____

_____

_____

_____

7. Discuss the technique of cognitive therapy and the goals related to this procedure. (pp. 795–796)

_____

_____

_____

_____

_____

8. Identify the various types of behavioral therapy techniques. Give definitions and examples.
   (Table 26–2, p. 795)

Behavioral Therapy Techniques

Type	Definition	Techniques

9. List the means of psychotherapy across the life span. (Table 26–3, p. 796)

Individual Psychotherapy across the Life Span

	Effective Psychotherapeutic Techniques	Nursing Challenges
Childhood		
Adolescence		
Early/middle adulthood		
Older adulthood		

10. List the issues and interventions related to therapeutic techniques used in mental health nursing.
    (Table 26–4, p. 802)

Therapeutic Techniques

Issue	Interventions

11. Discuss some of the factors that increase the likelihood of premature termination in a therapeutic relationship. (p. 804)

a. _____

b. _____

c. _____

d. _____

e. _____

f. _____

g. _____

h. _____

Case Study

Suggested answers for Case Studies are provided in the Answers section at the back of this Study Guide.

Scenario:
As the advanced-practice psychiatric nurse in a community mental health center, you have been assigned a client who looks very similar to a childhood friend, who was killed several years ago. The client is seeking counseling because of marital troubles.

1. Describe the goal of individual therapy

    _____

    _____

    _____

    _____

    _____

2. Once you recognize the client looks similar to your own family member, what should you be concerned about?

    _____

    _____

    _____

    _____

    _____

3. You decide the best course of action is to use cognitive therapy. Describe the concepts of cognitive therapy.

    _____

    _____

    _____

    _____

    _____

Self-Assessment Questions

Answers and rationales for Self-Assessment Questions are provided in the Answers section at the back of this Study Guide.

1. During an individual psychotherapy session, the advanced-practice psychiatric nurse, using the psychoanalytical approach, remains silent for a period of time. The client begins to talk about a topic new to their sessions. This is an example of:

    a.   Neutrality

    b.   Transference

    c.   Therapeutic alliance

    d.   Free association

2. During an individual psychotherapy session, the advanced-practice psychiatric nurse monitors herself and realizes that the client she is working with reminds her in some way of her childhood friend. This is an example of:

   a. Neutrality

   b. Countertransference

   c. Therapeutic alliance

   d. Free association

3. A new client is being seen in the community mental health clinic by the advanced-practice psychiatric nurse. Select all of the goals of psychotherapy for the client.

   a. Build a trust relationship

   b. Identify treatment goals

   c. Identify termination dates

   d. Assess the client's problems

   e. Remove distressful symptoms

   f. Support adaptive coping behaviors

   g. Promote optimal functioning

4. A client seeking relief from a fear of bridges is taken to a pedestrian crosswalk while being emotionally supported. This intervention is an example of:

   a. A nontherapeutic technique

   b. Systematic desensitization

   c. Flooding

   d. Aversion therapy

5. A child who is suspected of being sexually abused is being seen at the community mental health center. The therapist has given the child a doll. The purpose of the therapist's action is to:

   a. Allow the child to communicate symbolically

   b. Build a trusting relationship

   c. Accommodate for the shorter attention span of a child

   d. Preoccupy the child's time until therapy begins

6. An adolescent client in the community mental health center says, "I have to tell you something, but you have to promise you won't tell anyone else." The advanced-practice psychiatric nurse's most appropriate response is:

   a. "I promise."

   b. "I am bound by the nurse-client relationship to keep your comments private."

   c. "What is said in this room, stays in this room."

   d. "I cannot make that promise if it affects your safety or someone else's."

—NOTES—

CHAPTER 27

Group Therapy

This chapter discusses the role of the nurse in group therapy, including the theories and perspectives underlying group therapy. The types and various functions of groups that are used in the psychiatric setting are addressed, as well as how group therapy is implemented across the life span.

Reading Assignment

Prior to beginning this assignment, please read Chapter 27, "Group Therapy."

Activities

Using the content in the text, answer the following questions as clearly as you can and in your own words. Give examples, if appropriate, to help clarify the information in your answer.

1. Discuss aspects of Yalom's therapeutic factors for group therapy and give examples. (Table 27–2, p. 820)

a. _____

_____

_____

b. _____

_____

_____

c. _____

_____

_____

d. _____

_____

_____

e. _____

_____

_____

f. _____

_____

_____

g. _____

_____

_____

h. _____

_____

_____

i. _____

_____

_____

j. _____

_____

_____

k. _____

_____

_____

2. Explain "goodness of fit" in group therapy. (p. 821)

_____

_____

_____

_____

_____

3. Compare and contrast some of the advantages and disadvantages of group therapy. (pp. 820–821)

Advantages	**Disadvantages**

4. Identify the various models of group therapy. (pp. 821–823)

Models That May Be Used in Group Therapy

Model	How Used

5. Discuss the functions of a group leader. (p. 827)

- _____
- _____
- _____
- _____
- _____
- _____
- _____

6. List the two styles of group leadership and discuss the characteristics of each style. (Table 27–3, p. 827)

Summary of Characteristics of Group Leadership

Reflective	Authoritarian

7. Identify the types of groups used in group therapy, state their purposes, and give examples of each type. (Table 27–5, p. 829)

Types of Groups, Purposes, and Examples

Type of Group	Purpose(s)	Example(s)

8. Identify the issues related to group process across the life span. (Table 27–6, p. 834)

Group Therapy across the Life Span

Age Range	Issues That Are the Focus of Group Work

Case Study

Suggested answers for Case Studies are provided in the Answers section at the back of this Study Guide.

Scenario:
During group therapy, the following interaction takes place:

Member 1: I just don't know what to do. I have never been in a situation like this before. My husband wants to give up on our marriage, but I still love him.

Member 2: You'll make it through this. Don't give up.

Member 3: Yeah, if I can make it through a divorce and be as happy as I am, then you can too.

Member 4: We all go through rough times, maybe in different ways, but we all have our problems.

1. Which of Yalom's therapeutic factors for group therapy is Member 2 exemplifying?

_____

_____

_____

_____

_____

2. Member 3?

_____

_____

_____

_____

_____

3. Member 4?

_____

_____

_____

_____

_____

Self-Assessment Questions

Answers and rationales for Self-Assessment Questions are provided in the Answers section at the back of this Study Guide.

1. During group therapy, a male client speaks to a female client in a derogatory way and makes a sarcastic remark toward her about her "sloppiness." The group therapist analyzes this behavior as an example of which of Yalom's therapeutic factors for group therapy?

   a. Corrective recapitulation of the primary family

   b. Imitative behavior

   c. Group cohesiveness

   d. Catharsis

2. During group therapy, a male client speaks to a female client in a derogatory way and makes a sarcastic remark toward her about her "sloppiness." Which of the following interventions by the group therapist is most appropriate?

   a. "I am wondering if anyone noticed you spoke to her like you speak to your wife."

   b. "Sir, we must be respectful at all times in group."

   c. "Why do you suppose you spoke to her that way?"

   d. "I find it very uncomfortable when I hear you treat others in this way."

3. A group member states in the fifth meeting of the group, "You guys are the best. I was sure no one would understand what I was going through." This is an example of which of Yalom's therapeutic factors for group therapy?

   a. Instillation of hope

   b. Universality

   c. Catharsis

   d. Imparting information

4. During the orientation phase of the group therapy session, the members of the group have the following interchange:

   Member A: As the leader, you just think you know it all.

   Member B: Yeah, I bet you have never been in our shoes.

   Member C: You get to go home at night and relax. We have to stay and work on our problems. How fair is that?

   This interchange is an example of which of Yalom's therapeutic factors for group therapy?

   a. Universality

   b. Group cohesiveness

   c. Catharsis

   d. Imparting information

5. Following the death of her husband, a widow joins a group of other widowers. The type of group that she is joining is likely:

    a. A social group

    b. A self-help group

    c. A symptom management group

    d. A task group

6. An inpatient group on medication management on a psychiatric unit is held every other day. Which type of group is this most likely to be?

    a. Psychoeducational

    b. Experimental

    c. Educational

    d. Psychoanalytical

7. A client with bipolar disorder is actively hallucinating and frequently pacing the halls of the psychiatric unit of the hospital. In which of the following groups should the client participate?

    a. A highly structured task group

    b. A self-help group

    c. A psychoeducational group

    d. Group is not appropriate for this client at this time.

8. When planning a psychoeducational group therapy session, the nurse should make which of the following plans?

    a. Limit the size to one to three clients

    b. Set up the room in rows

    c. Provide desks

    d. Select a closed room

9. Educational preparation for a nurse group therapist is:

    a. An RN license

    b. An associate's degree

    c. A master's degree and supervised practiced as a group leader

    d. A doctorate degree in counseling

10. During group therapy, a client asks the nurse group leader for advice on how to handle the stress of her new job. The best approach for the leader is to:

    a. Answer her question directly

    b. Enlist the other group members to respond

    c. Encourage the client to speak to her after group

    d. Use silence

CHAPTER 28

Familial Systems and Family Therapy

This chapter looks at the evolution of families across the life span and the role of the specialist and advanced-practice psychiatric nurse in caring for all types of families. Communication—incongruent, impaired, and congruent—is also addressed.

Reading Assignment

Prior to beginning this assignment, please read Chapter 28, "Familial Systems and Family Therapy."

Activities

Using the content in the text, answer the following questions as clearly as you can and in your own words. Give examples, if appropriate, to help clarify the information in your answer.

1. Discuss the major family subsystems and their composition. Provide examples of each type. (Table 28–1, p. 851)

Major Family Structures

Type	Composition	Example

2. Discuss family functions that are critical to the well-being of family members, according to Epstein and Bishop. (p. 853)

a. _____

b. _____

c. _____

d. _____

e. _____

3. Discuss the major family tasks according to Duvall. Provide examples of each major task. (Table 28–2, p. 852)

Discussion of Tasks   **Examples**

a. _____   _____

b. _____   _____

c. _____   _____

d. _____   _____

e. _____   _____

f. _____   _____

g. _____   _____

h. _____   _____

4. Identify the areas of family function that influence healthy outcomes in times of crisis or change. Supply definitions and examples. (p. 853)

Areas of Family Function That Help to Determine Healthy Outcomes in Times of Crisis/Change

Area	Definition	Examples

5. Discuss how general systems theory can be applied to families. (pp. 853–855)

_____

_____

_____

_____

_____

6. Differentiate among incongruent, impaired, and congruent communication, giving examples from the content in the text. (p. 855)

_____

_____

_____

_____

_____

7. List the ways for health care providers to develop culturally sensitive family interventions as suggested by Odell et al. Give examples that you have observed in clinical experiences. (p. 857)

- _____
  _____
- _____
  _____
- _____
  _____
- _____
  _____
- _____
  _____
- _____
  _____

8. Identify the characteristics of functional and dysfunctional familial systems. (Table 28–4, p. 861)

Characteristics of Functional and Dysfunctional Familial Systems

Component	Functional Families	Dysfunctional Families

9. Identify the stages of family development and related tasks according to Howell. Provide examples. (Table 28–5, p. 862)

Evolution of the Family: Developmental Stages

Stage	Task(s)

10. Identify the components of family assessment in structural therapy and the associated interventions. (Table 28–6, p. 866)

Components of Family Assessment of Structural Therapy

Component	Intervention

Case Study

Suggested answers for Case Studies are provided in the Answers section at the back of this Study Guide.

Scenario:
As part of an adolescent inpatient treatment plan, the family is brought in for family therapy. During the initial meeting of the family, the father gives his son a hug but then states jokingly, "I sure haven't missed having your loud music blaring all over the house." During the interview, the mother says, "If your father had paid more attention to you on weekends, we wouldn't be here today." To which the father says, "If you wouldn't baby the kids so much, we wouldn't be here today."

1. What kind of messages is the family displaying?

_____

_____

_____

_____

_____

2. Describe the role of the therapist when working with the family.

_____

_____

_____

_____

_____

Self-Assessment Questions

Answers and rationales for Self-Assessment Questions are provided in the Answers section at the back of this Study Guide.

1. An adolescent girl is observed sitting on her father's lap while he strokes her hair. Although no sexual abuse is suspected, the nurse analyzes this behavior within the family as:
   a. Double-bind message
   b. Boundary issues
   c. Marital schism
   d. Open family system

2. During a divorce proceeding, the court orders the children to go into counseling because of the turmoil of the parents' continued fighting. The 10-year-old son states, "When I am at my mom's house, she always asks if my dad has any girlfriends over. When I am at my dad's house, he tells me I don't have to follow Mom's rules." This is an example of which family dynamic?

    a. Double-bind messages
    b. Equilibrium
    c. Feedback
    d. Marital schism

3. The mother of a daughter being sexually abused by the mother's common-law husband is aware of the abuse. The mother does not act upon her awareness of the situation until the daughter seeks help from the school counselor. When confronted with the situation, the mother admits she knew it was going on but didn't stop it. This is an example of which family dynamic?

    a. Open system
    b. Marital skew
    c. Scapegoating
    d. Enmeshment

4. An adolescent is hospitalized for depression and suicidal ideation. During family therapy, the following interaction takes place:

    Dad: Things have been going from bad to worse. He is not helping by being in here. This will cost us a lot of money we could use elsewhere.

    Mother: He has always been an unruly boy. He has caused me a lot of stress.

    This interchange suggests which of the following family dynamics?

    a. Relational resilience
    b. Scapegoating
    c. Marital skew
    d. Enmeshment

5. Select all of the following groups that constitute a family structure.

    a. Two parents never before married with two biological children
    b. Single parent living with great aunt
    c. Boyfriend, girlfriend, and child living together in a single-room dwelling
    d. Remarried couple with four stepchildren
    e. Homosexual couple sharing a mortgage

6. A 30-year-old employed son still lives at home with his family. His mother continues to do his laundry and fix his meals. His chores are limited to taking out the trash. He pays no rent. Which of the following family tasks has this family not achieved?

    a. Allocation of resources

    b. Socialization of members

    c. Maintenance of motivation

    d. Placement of members into society

7. During family therapy, a couple is arguing about the discipline of the children. The father turns to the nurse therapist and states, "What do you think about her letting the kids stay up so late?" This interaction is consistent with which family dynamic?

    a. Disengagement

    b. Triangulation

    c. Enmeshment

    d. Double-bind message

8. A blended family of stepparents and stepchildren are preparing to celebrate the first family holiday together. One child states, "We always go to church on Christmas Eve." Another child says, "Well, I have always gone to my grandma's house on Christmas Eve." The father says, "I think we can arrange to do both." The father's comments are an example of which major task of stepfamilies?

    a. Resolving issues from the previous marriage

    b. Forming new relationships

    c. Reconstructing roles

    d. Establishing new rituals

9. A neighborhood boy raped a young girl after school. The girl's family is traumatized and enters into family therapy. The mother states, "We are just devastated, but we will do whatever we need to do to support our daughter and move on." The father states, "I am just at a loss to know what to do. Our daughter's well-being is of the utmost importance. Whatever it takes, we'll do." These comments are most closely associated with which of the following dynamics?

    a. Scapegoating

    b. Triangulation

    c. Relational resilience

    d. Marital skew

CHAPTER 29

Psychopharmacologic Therapy

This chapter begins with a discussion of the structures of the brain that are affected by the use of psychotropic medication. A nursing process approach is used to help the nurse to plan care for patients receiving medications.

Reading Assignment

Prior to beginning this assignment, please read Chapter 29, "Psychopharmacologic Therapy."

Activities

Using the content in the text, answer the following questions as clearly as you can and in your own words. Give examples, if appropriate, to help clarify the information in your answer.

1. Draw the synaptic gap and indicate how four major neurotransmitters effect the function of the brain. (pp. 881–883)

    a. _____

    b. _____

    c. _____

    d. _____

2. Discuss factors influencing the intensity and duration of drug effects. (pp. 884–885)

   a. _____

   b. _____

   c. _____

   d. _____

3. Differentiate among steady state, half-life, and clearance as they relate to the administration of medication. (p. 885)

   Steady state_____

   _____

   _____

   Half-life_____

   _____

   _____

   Clearance _____

   _____

   _____

4. Fill in the correct information. (Table 29–12, p. 903)

   Extrapyramidal Side Effects from Antipsychotic Medications

	Acute Dystonia	Akathisia	Akinesia	Dyskinesia	Dystonia	Tardive Dyskinesia
Manifestations						
Onset						
Treatment						

5. Fill in the correct information. (Table 29–14, p. 905)

   Adverse Effects Associated with Antiparkinsonian Medications for Extrapyramidal Side Effects

System	Common Side Effects	Less Common Side Effects

6. Fill in the correct information. (Table 29–15, p. 906)

Adverse Effects Associated with Antipsychotics

System	Common Side Effects	Less Common Side Effects

7. Fill in the correct information. (Table 29–19, p. 914)

Adverse Effects Associated with Sedatives and Hypnotics

System	Common Side Effects	Less Common Side Effects
BENZODIAZEPINES		
NONBARBITURATES		
BARBITURATES		

8. Discuss the measures that are recommended, before a client is started on tricyclic antidepressants. (p. 917)

   a. _____

   b. _____

   c. _____

9. Discuss some of the factors that contribute to nonadherence to medication regimens in older adults. (p. 924)

   • _____

   • _____

   • _____

   • _____

   • _____

   • _____

   • _____

   • _____

10. List current FDA categories for drug use in pregnancy. (Table 29–21, p. 921)

   • _____

   • _____

   • _____

   • _____

11. Discuss the guidelines that should be used for enhancing medication adherence. (Table 29–22, p. 925)

   • _____

   • _____

   • _____

   • _____

   • _____

   • _____

Case Study

Suggested answers for Case Studies are provided in the Answers section at the back of this Study Guide.

Scenario:

A young man is brought by his roommate to the emergency department. His symptoms include unusual sleepiness, muscle twitching, staggered walk, and increased deep tendon reflexes. Earlier in the day he ran a 10-kilometer race for the first time. The day is hot and humid. Medications include Eskalith.

1. What lab test is essential to obtain immediately?

   _____

   _____

   _____

   _____

   _____

2. His lithium level returns as 1.9 mEq/L. Interpret this lab value.

   _____

   _____

   _____

   _____

   _____

3. When told of his lithium level, he states, "But I am taking my medication just as it is prescribed. I didn't take any more or any less. Just like I always do." Could this statement be true in light of the lab value? Why or why not?

   _____

   _____

   _____

   _____

4. What further teaching needs to be done with the client?

_____

_____

_____

_____

_____

Self-Assessment Questions

Answers and rationales for Self-Assessment Questions are provided in the Answers section at the back of this Study Guide.

1. A client is taking a monoamine oxidase inhibitor (MAO). Which comment by the client would indicate that the nurse needs to teach the client further about the medication the client is taking?

    a.   "I can't wait to bite into that orange I have saved for my snack."

    b.   "I ordered a banana for breakfast tomorrow."

    c.   "The apples here are delicious."

    d.   "I had tomatoes on my salad."

2. A male client taking trazodone (Desyrel) calls the community mental health clinic to cancel his appointment. The nurse asks him why he needs to cancel. Embarrassed, he states he has an erection that will not go away. The nurse's most appropriate response is:

    a.   "I understand. Can we reschedule for next week?"

    b.   "That is a problem."

    c.   "Do not take any more of your medication and come to the emergency department right away."

    d.   "I still expect you to make your appointment on time."

3. A client who has started on an antidepressant complains of a dry mouth. The nurse's most appropriate response is to:

    a.   Call the physician immediately

    b.   Offer sugarless gum or candy or sips of water

    c.   Assess blood pressure

    d.   Interpret the behavior as attention seeking

4. A client on an monoamine oxidase inhibitor (MAOI) complains of a headache and nausea. The nurse's most appropriate response is to:

    a.   Take the blood pressure and call the doctor

    b.   Assess for further flu-like symptoms

    c.   Give a prn antiparkinsonian agent

    d.   Give prn aspirin

5. A client on an antipsychotic medication gets out of bed as soon as breakfast arrives in the dayroom. Halfway to the eating area, the client puts his hand to his head and grabs the wall to steady himself. The nurse's most appropriate interpretation of this behavior is:

    a. The client is seeking attention.

    b. The client should be assessed for orthostatic hypotension.

    c. The client has tardive dyskinesia.

    d. The client's behavior is a precursor to oculogyric crisis.

6. A client has been started on an antipsychotic medication. On a medication follow-up at the community mental health clinic, the nurse notices the client wiggling her tongue. What interpretation of the client's behavior is most important to assess further?

    a. The client might be using passive-aggressive behaviors.

    b. The client is seeking attention.

    c. The client will need a complete blood count.

    d. The client may have early signs of tardive dyskinesia.

7. The community mental health nurse observes the following behaviors in an elderly client who is taking an antipsychotic medication: drooling and pill-rolling hand tremors. The nurse's best response is to:

    a. Refer the client to a neurologist for evaluation

    b. Check for a prn order for Cogentin

    c. Assess the client's diet

    d. Ask the client to wipe his mouth

8. A client who has been taking a selective serotonin reuptake inhibitor comes into the mental health clinic complaining of feeling lightheaded and sleepy and has both a headache and nausea. Which question by the nurse is most appropriate to ask?

    a. "When was the last time you took your medication?"

    b. "Do you remember when we talked about somatic complaints and depression?"

    c. "Have you been around anyone with the flu?"

    d. "Could you be pregnant?"

9. Client A's eyes are rotated upward and laterally. Client B complains of feeling dizzy when he gets out of bed. Client C complains of blurred vision. Client D complains of being sleepy. Which client must the nurse notify the doctor of immediately?

    a. Client A

    b. Client B

    c. Client C

    d. Client D

10. A client on lithium has a blood level of 1.8 mEq/L. The nursing diagnosis with the highest priority is:

    a. Risk for injury related to manic hyperactivity

    b. Risk for injury related to toxicity

    c. Risk for activity intolerance related to side effects

    d. Knowledge deficit related to medication

CHAPTER 30

Electroconvulsive, Other Biological (Somatic), and Complementary Therapies

Electroconvulsive and other biological therapies, such as vagus nerve stimulation, transmagnetic stimulation, and complementary therapies such as acupuncture, light therapy, and massage therapy, are discussed in this chapter. The nursing process approach is used to determine the nurse's role in administering these therapies.

Reading Assignment

Prior to beginning this assignment, please read Chapter 30, "Electroconvulsive, Other Biological (Somatic), and Complementary Therapies."

Activities

Using the content in the text, answer the following questions as clearly as you can and in your own words. Give examples, if appropriate, to help clarify the information in your answer.

1. Discuss the biological therapies that have been used historically for treating mental disorders. (pp. 937–939)

   a. Psychosurgery_____

   _____

   b. Hydrotherapy _____

   _____

   c. Convulsive therapies _____

   _____

   l. Insulin-shock therapy_____

   _____

2. Metrazol _____

_____

_____

3. Electroshock therapy _____

_____

_____

4. Vagus nerve stimulation _____

_____

_____

5. Transcranial magnetic stimulation _____

_____

_____

6. Deep brain stimulation _____

_____

_____

2. Give examples of individuals who are good candidates for electroconvulsive therapy. (p. 939)

- _____
- _____
- _____
- _____
- _____
- _____

3. Fill in the correct information. (Table 30–2, p. 941)

Major Biological Responses to ECT

Major Physiological Responses to ECT	
Cardiovascular	**Cerebral**
Theories of Neurobiological Effects of ECT	
Neurochemical	**Neurophysiological**

4. Discuss the role of the nurse in caring for the client undergoing ECT treatment. (pp. 944–945)

   a. _____

   b. _____

   c. _____

   d. _____

5. Discuss pretreatment nursing care for ECT. (p. 945)

   a. _____

   b. _____

   c. _____

   d. _____

   e. _____

   f. _____

6. Discuss the other biological and complementary therapies that are used with clients with psychiatric conditions. (pp. 951–954)

   Light therapy _____

   _____

   _____

   Acupuncture _____

   _____

   _____

   Aromatherapy _____

   _____

   _____

   Massage therapy _____

   _____

   _____

Case Study

Suggested answers for Case Studies are provided in the Answers section at the back of this Study Guide.

Scenario:
A client is diagnosed with seasonal affective disorder and is to be started on light therapy.

1. Prepare a teaching plan for this client.

   _____

   _____

   _____

   _____

   _____

2. What assessments would be important to complete with this client at 7 days, 2 weeks, and routinely thereafter?

    _____

    _____

    _____

    _____

    _____

3. What is the theoretical basis for light therapy?

    _____

    _____

    _____

    _____

    _____

Self-Assessment Questions

Answers and rationales for Self-Assessment Questions are provided in the Answers section at the back of this Study Guide.

1. An elderly client is being prepared for his first electroconvulsive therapy treatment. He asks, "How is this treatment going to make me feel better?" The nurse's best response is:

    a. "Although it isn't exactly known how it works, research indicates it improves brain functioning for people with depression."

    b. "It works by calming the brain cells."

    c. "It satisfies the need to be punished by individuals who feel a lot of guilt."

    d. "I don't know, but it works."

2. Of the following clients, which is the most likely to be receiving ECT?

    a. A client with bipolar disorder in the manic phase

    b. A client with cyclothymia

    c. An elderly client with depression and abnormal liver function tests

    d. A client with schizophrenia who is hallucinating

3. Which of the statements by a client undergoing ECT treatment needs further teaching?

    a. "I should be able to eat shortly after the treatment."

    b. "Someone will help me to breathe during the procedure."

    c. "I will lose the memories of my childhood."

    d. "I need to sign a consent to have this done."

4. In preparing a client for the first ECT treatment, the nurse identifies which of the following goals as the highest priority?

   a. The client will experience minimal anxiety about the ECT procedure.

   b. The client will get approval from family members.

   c. The client will acknowledge that ECT is the preferred treatment.

   d. The client will state his need to have treatment.

5. At the community mental health clinic, the office manager has placed lavender room fresheners in the waiting room and throughout the office area. When a co-worker asks the advanced-practice nurse the reason for the change in the office environment, the nurse's best response is that:

   a. Using lavender essence as aromatherapy has calming or tranquilizing effects.

   b. It is her favorite color.

   c. The office needed some sprucing up.

   d. It helps the clients keep their minds off of their problems.

6. A firefighter whose work shift varies from days to nights on a regular basis complains of fatigue, irritability, and depression. In analyzing the firefighter's complaints, the nurse's most appropriate interpretation is that:

   a. The firefighter may have interrupted circadian rhythms.

   b. The firefighter should be assessed for seasonal affective disorder.

   c. The firefighter should be assessed for sleep medication.

   d. The firefighter has abnormal melatonin levels.

7. An elderly client is being prepared for his first electroconvulsive therapy treatment. He asks, "Is this some new-fangled experiment?" The nurse's best response is:

   a. "Successful ECT treatment has been around for about 60 years."

   b. "It is a recently devised treatment for depression."

   c. "Only certain clients with depression have been allowed to have ECT since federal guidelines have been put in place."

   d. "ECT has recently been found to be more effective and safer than antidepressant medications."

—NOTES—

CHAPTER 31

Crisis Intervention Management: The Role of Adaptation

In this chapter, the difference between maturational crisis and situational crisis is defined, and the coping mechanisms that are used in response to stress are identified. The role of the nurse in caring for patients in crisis is also addressed.

Reading Assignment

Prior to beginning this assignment, please read Chapter 31, "Crisis Intervention Management: The Role of Adaptation."

Activities

Using the content in the text, answer the following questions as clearly as you can and in your own words. Give examples, if appropriate, to help clarify the information in your answer.

1. Identify Erik Erikson's stages of development and responses to crisis situations. Give examples of each. (Table 31–1, p. 964)

Maturational Crises: Erikson's Eight Stages of Development

Primary Developmental Task	Sources of Maladaptive Responses to Crises	Example

2. Explain the difference between situational crisis and maturational crisis. Give examples. (pp. 964–967)

Situational crisis _____

_____

_____

_____

_____

Examples _____

_____

_____

_____

_____

Maturational crisis _____

_____

_____

_____

_____

Examples _____

_____

_____

_____

_____

3. Differentiate among primary appraisal, secondary appraisal, and reappraisal. Give examples. (p. 968)

Primary appraisal _____

_____

_____

Secondary appraisal _____

_____

_____

Reappraisal _____

_____

_____

4. Discuss the factors that determine how families handle stressful situations according to Caplan. (p. 973)

a. _____

b. _____

c. _____

d. _____

e. _____

Case Study

Suggested answers for Case Studies are provided in the Answers section at the back of this Study Guide.

Scenario:
A small town was devastated by a major tornado. Many of the residents lost their homes and all of their possessions. Fortunately, no deaths were reported. As part of the disaster response team, you are meeting with families to determine their needs. While helping to obtain vision and medication prescriptions for a middle-aged woman, she states, "I am just in shock. I don't have anything. All of my children's pictures are gone. My grandmother's ring is gone. I don't have a job, I suppose, because it is gone, too. Where will the kids go to school? How will they get there?"

1. Does the resident require primary or secondary appraisal?

   _____

   _____

   _____

   _____

   _____

2. What subtype of appraisal is the resident describing?

   _____

   _____

   _____

   _____

   _____

3. What is the goal of crisis intervention for this resident?

   _____

   _____

   _____

   _____

   _____

Self-Assessment Questions

Answers and rationales for Self-Assessment Questions are provided in the Answers section at the back of this Study Guide.

1. Which of the following is most closely associated with crisis intervention?
   a. Therapy for an eating disorder
   b. A self-help group such as Alcoholics Anonymous
   c. An anger management group
   d. Support following a rape

2. A teenager becomes pregnant and tells her parents, who react with shock and anger. The family accepts a referral for family counseling. Although they have been challenged, the family states at the termination of the sessions, "We feel like we are closer as a family now." The appropriate interpretation of this statement is:

   a. The family is using denial.

   b. Families in crisis can develop new coping mechanisms.

   c. The family has learned to say what the family members think the therapist wants to hear.

   d. The birth of the baby has changed the family's perspective.

3. A college student is involved in a serious monogamous relationship for the first time. This is an example of which of the following developmental tasks of maturational crises?

   a. Trust vs. mistrust

   b. Autonomy vs. shame/doubt

   c. Identify vs. role confusion

   d. Intimacy vs. isolation

4. Three of the following examples are of conditions that need to be present to produce a crisis. Which condition is not necessary for crisis development?

   a. A fire in one's home

   b. Anxiety over loss of possessions in a fire

   c. Crying when remembering a fire

   d. Accepting assistance from a community agency

5. Which of the following situations is an example of a situational, interpersonal crisis?

   a. Fire

   b. Riot

   c. Amputation

   d. Death of a spouse

6. An example of the generativity of the middle adulthood developmental stage is:

   a. Teaching religious classes at one's place of worship

   b. Getting married

   c. Attending college to learn a profession

   d. Following the posted speed limit

7. A client is being seen for crisis intervention after being in a plane crash in which most passengers were killed. The client states, "Why me? Why did I live and the guy next to me didn't? Should I be doing something special?" This comment reflects which psychological response to a disaster?

   a. Psychic numbing

   b. Death guilt

   c. Death anxiety

   d. Struggle for significance

8. A client whose husband recently died cries every day for long periods of time. She has neglected her activities of daily living such as bathing and eating. Which of the following nursing diagnoses is most appropriate for this client?

   a. Fear

   b. Disturbed body image

   c. Ineffective coping

   d. Ineffective home maintenance

9. A client unable to cope with the effects of a tornado and who is struggling to keep her family together is experiencing which of the following types of crisis?

   a. Developmental

   b. Situational

   c. Social

   d. Maturational

10. The advanced-practice psychiatric nurse who practices crisis intervention understands that the goal of crisis intervention is different from the goal of group therapy in that crisis intervention:

   a. Is focused on reaching at least the pre-crisis level of functioning

   b. Defines the psychopathology of the situation

   c. Has as a goal the client's self-actualization

   d. Provides for the enactment of the family dynamics

—NOTES—

CHAPTER 32

Milieu Therapy/ Hospital-Based Care

The term *milieu therapy* is readily used in the mental health arena. This chapter gives an explicit accounting of all aspects of this mode of treatment, including the specific tools used in mental health nursing to provide comprehensive care to clients.

Reading Assignment

Prior to beginning this assignment, please read Chapter 32, "Milieu Therapy/Hospital-Based Care."

Activities

Using the content in the text, answer the following questions as clearly as you can and in your own words. Give examples, if appropriate, to help clarify the information in your answer.

1. Identify the eight concepts and principles of the "new" milieu therapy, giving examples of each. (pp. 987–993)

Concepts and Principles of Milieu Therapy in a New Era

Concept/Principle	Examples

2. With use of assertive community treatment and intensive case management, improvement in clients can be seen in the following areas of treatment outcomes: (p. 998)

   a. _____

   b. _____

   c. _____

   d. _____

3. Examples of structure in the mental health environment include: (pp. 990–991)

   a. _____

   b. _____

   c. _____

   d. _____

4. Give examples of nursing interventions that promote involvement in milieu therapy. (p. 991)

   • _____

   • _____

   • _____

   • _____

   • _____

5. Document the elements of milieu therapy across the life span. (Table 32–1, pp. 994–995)

Milieu Elements and Interventions across the Life Span

	Child	Adolescent	Adult	Older Adult

6. Discuss the role of the nurse in milieu therapy. (pp. 996–997)

a. _____

b. _____

c. _____

d. _____

e. _____

f. _____

g. _____

h. _____

Case Study

Suggested answers for Case Studies are provided in the Answers section at the back of this Study Guide.

Scenario:

An acute psychiatric unit is designed as a locked unit and has several interdisciplinary therapeutic groups each day. It includes a group meeting in the morning that orients newly admitted clients to the expectations of the unit. A recreational therapy group is offered, and two group therapy sessions are offered at specified times each day. A cognitive therapy group that focuses on adherence to medications or anger management is provided every other day. Meals are served on the unit in the common room with small tables that seat four people. Snacks and refreshments are available throughout the day and evening. Each client has a double room shared with a roommate, and each room has its own bathroom with shower.

1. Which of the concepts and principles of milieu therapy can be identified in this psychiatric unit?

_____

_____

_____

_____

_____

2. What is the role of the psychiatric nurse during the containment period?

_____

_____

_____

_____

_____

Self-Assessment Questions

Answers and rationales for Self-Assessment Questions are provided in the Answers section at the back of this Study Guide.

1. A client is hospitalized to an acute psychiatric unit for suicidal ideation. Which element of a holding environment is the most important for this client?

   a. Self-understanding

   b. Socialization

   c. Structure

   d. Safety

2. The morning community group activity on the psychiatric unit reviews the time of the scheduled activities throughout the day. Which element of a holding environment is most closely associated with this activity?

   a. Socialization

   b. Structure

   c. Support

   d. Self-understanding

3. In the remodeling of a psychiatric unit, decisions were made to install breakaway showerheads and towel racks. The nursing diagnosis that prompted this decision is:

   a. Ineffective home maintenance

   b. Self-care deficit

   c. Ineffective coping

   d. Risk for violence directed at self

4. A client is placed in a seclusion room because of imminent risk of harming another. The appropriate basis for this decision is:

   a. Secluding a client punishes the client for unsocialized behavior.

   b. Seclusion rooms are a form of aversion therapy.

   c. The environment is used to provide protection for the client and others.

   d. The client needs to learn issues of power and control.

5. A child in the child/adolescent section of a psychiatric unit wants to play a board game. The other children want to toss the beanbag. When the child who wants to play the board game does not get his way, he takes the beanbags and hides them in the dayroom. Rather than intervene, the nurse allows the other kids to voice their displeasure. The nurse used which concept of milieu therapy?

   a. Peer pressure can be useful and powerful.

   b. The nurse wanted to assess whether any of the children would act out.

   c. The nurse determined that the behavior was inconsequential.

   d. The nurse was concerned the group would direct its anger toward the nurse.

6. Which of the following initial statements by the admitting nurse to the client upon arrival to the psychiatric unit is most therapeutic?

    a. "I see your name is Pat. I have a sister named Pat."

    b. "I'll take you to your room and I'll be in to see you in an hour or so."

    c. "My name is Kristi and I am your nurse today. Let's sit down here and talk."

    d. "Why are you here in the hospital?"

—NOTES—

CHAPTER 33

Home- and Community-Based Care

This chapter focuses on home and community-based care of persons with psychiatric disorders. Several resources are identified that offer care to all age-groups. The issues of homelessness and alcohol and substance abuse are also addressed.

Reading Assignment

Prior to beginning this assignment, please read Chapter 33, "Home- and Community-Based Care."

Activities

Using the content in the text, answer the following questions as clearly as you can and in your own words. Give examples, if appropriate, to help clarify the information in your answer.

1. Differentiate among primary, secondary, and tertiary prevention, and give examples of each. (p. 1009)

Levels of Care in Community Mental Health

Level of Care	Definition	Example
Primary		
Secondary		
Tertiary		

2. Identify the common diagnoses that can be treated using partial hospitalization and the treatment methods used. (Table 33–1, p. 1010)

Partial Hospitalization across the Life Span

Age-Group	Common Diagnosis	Therapeutic Modality(ies)

3. Explain the nurse's role in palliative or end-of-life care with individuals of all ages. (Table 33–2, p. 1014)

Hospice Care Issues across the Life Span

Age-Group	Response to Death and Dying	Nursing Implication(s)

4. List the educational programs that are provided by community mental health programs. (Table 33–3, p. 1015)

Educational Programs Provided by Community Mental Health Centers

Population Served	Programs

Case Study

Suggested answers for Case Studies are provided in the Answers section at the back of this Study Guide.

Scenario:
After discharge from an acute psychiatric care facility, clients are instructed to come to an outpatient clinic to be seen by the advanced-practice psychiatric nurse. The purpose of the visit is to monitor medication adherence.

1. What level of care in the community is the advanced-practice psychiatric nurse fulfilling?

_____

_____

_____

_____

_____

Self-Assessment Questions

Answers and rationales for Self-Assessment Questions are provided in the Answers section at the back of this Study Guide.

1. As the community mental health nurse in a specified area, the nurse recognizes the importance of early detection of clients with schizophrenia. The rationale for early detection is:
   a. The course of illness is affected by the quality of care in the early stages of the disorder.
   b. Long-term planning is more effective when case loads can be predicted.
   c. Budget planning is contingent on case load.
   d. Support services can be instituted.

2. Three of the following are case manager roles of the psychiatric–mental health nurse. Identify the activity that is not a role of the psychiatric–mental health nurse.

    a.   Conduct physical, spiritual, psychological, and cultural assessments of consumers

    b.   Collaborate with family members of consumers

    c.   Monitor client responses to medications

    d.   Transport consumers to dental appointments

3. A strategy most closely associated with primary prevention is:

    a.   Teaching a class on helpful coping strategies in a health class in a high school

    b.   Counseling a family that has just lost their home in a fire

    c.   Teaching a depressed client when and how to take her antidepressant medication

    d.   Facilitating anger management classes at a group home for individuals with mental illnesses

4. An activity most closely associated with secondary prevention is:

    a.   Teaching assertiveness skills at the local high school

    b.   Leading a self-help group for recent widows

    c.   Teaching anger management skills to a client with bipolar disorder

    d.   Providing community mental health services after discharge

5. A client with chronic schizophrenia is in need of psychiatric care. He lives alone, adheres to his medication schedule some of the time but not always, and hears voices a couple of times a week. Which type of service is most appropriate for this client?

    a.   Locked, intensive, psychiatric unit

    b.   General psychiatric unit in a hospital

    c.   Day treatment program

    d.   He is not in need of services.

6. Of the following, select all of the programs provided by community mental health centers.

    a.   Stress management

    b.   Medication management

    c.   Individual counseling

    d.   Suicide precautions

    e.   Psychological testing

—NOTES—

CHAPTER 34

Psychosocial Care in Medical-Surgical Settings

It is very important for nurses in the medical-surgical setting to be aware of the psychosocial needs of clients in their care. This chapter provides background guidance on how to deliver effective psychosocial nursing care in these settings.

Reading Assignment

Prior to beginning this assignment, please read Chapter 34, "Psychosocial Care in Medical-Surgical Settings."

Activities

Using the content in the text, answer the following questions as clearly as you can and in your own words. Give examples, if appropriate, to help clarify the information in your answer.

1. Discuss some of the types of clients in a medical-surgical setting for whom providing nursing care may prove to be challenging. (pp. 1026–1030)

   _____

   _____

   _____

2. What are some of the feelings that are generated in the nurse when the client is angry or demanding? (p. 1027)

   _____

   _____

   _____

   _____

   _____

3. How can feelings generated in the nurse by an angry client be effectively managed? (p. 1028)

_____

_____

_____

_____

_____

4. List some of the dos and don'ts for dealing with an angry client. Give examples of each. (Table 34–1, p. 1028)

Dos and Don'ts for Coping with the Angry Client

What to Do	Why	Example

What Not to Do	Why

5. List some of the dos and don'ts for dealing with a demanding client. Give examples. (Table 34–2, p. 1029)

Dos and Don'ts for Coping with the Demanding Client

What to Do	Why	Example

What Not to Do	Why

6. Discuss the stages of grief according to Kübler-Ross. Give examples of each. (Table 34–3, p. 1030)

Kübler-Ross's Five Stages of Grief Applied to the Medical-Surgical Client

Stage	Client Behavior	Example

7. Develop a care plan for a client with AIDS delirium. (p. 1035)

   a. _____

   b. _____

   c _____

   d. _____

   e. _____

8. Discuss major psychosocial stressors for poststroke clients. (p. 1037)

   a. _____

   b. _____

   c. _____

   d. _____

   e. _____

   f. _____

   g. _____

9. Describe the major nursing diagnoses related to clients who are experiencing psychosocial stressors. (p. 1039)

   a. _____

   b. _____

   c. _____

   d. _____

   e. _____

   f. _____

Case Study

Suggested answers for Case Studies are provided in the Answers section at the back of this Study Guide.

Scenario:
A client has just been diagnosed with terminal cancer. The family has been told by the physician that there is nothing that can be done except to make the client comfortable. Initially the wife states, "That can't be. We just got back from vacation and he was just fine." The next day the son walks into the nurses' station and demands to know who is taking care of his father. "He hasn't been given anything to eat today. I want to know what is going on here. Isn't this place supposed to be a hospital?"

1. What stage of grief does the wife indicate by her statements?

   _____

   _____

   _____

   _____

   _____

2. What stage of grief does the son indicate by his statements?

   _____

   _____

   _____

   _____

   _____

3. What is a therapeutic response by the nurse to the son?

   _____

   _____

   _____

   _____

   _____

Self-Assessment Questions

Answers and rationales for Self-Assessment Questions are provided in the Answers section at the back of this Study Guide.

1. On a busy medical-surgical floor of a hospital, a client demands that his pain medication be brought immediately. He yells and makes a fist as he talks. Which of the following statements by the nurse is most therapeutic?

   a. "I can see you are very angry about this."

   b. "As soon as I can, I will!"

   c. "Yelling isn't helping any."

   d. "I am doing the best I can."

2. Three of the following strategies are helpful when coping with an angry client. Select the strategy that is not helpful when coping with an angry client.

   a. Touching the client

   b. Watching the client's body language

   c. Allowing the client to express his feelings

   d. Keeping calm

3. Three of the following strategies are helpful with coping with a demanding client. Select the strategy that is not helpful when coping with a demanding client.

   a. Setting limits

   b. Keeping promises

   c. Limiting complaints to one or two statements

   d. Recognizing that the client is feeling fearful, anxious, or angry

4. The mother of a teenager killed in a car accident has just arrived at the emergency department. The nurse has to inform the mother of the death. Based on Kübler-Ross's five stages of grief, the nurse would expect the mother to exhibit behaviors consistent with which of the following stages?

   a. Acceptance

   b. Anger

   c. Bargaining

   d. Denial

5. The husband of a woman dying of cancer has been involved with her hospice care for several weeks. The hospice nurse has taught him the physiological signs of impending death. At the moment of death, the husband picks up his wife's hand and kisses her warmly on the cheek while saying, "I love you." Which stage of Kübler-Ross's stages of grieving is consistent with the behavior of the husband?

   a. Denial

   b. Bargaining

   c. Depression

   d. Acceptance

—NOTES—

UNIT 4

Advancing Psychiatric Nursing Practice

Chapter 35   Psychiatric Consultation-Liaison Nursing

Chapter 36   Psychiatric Nursing Research

Chapter 37   The Future of Psychiatric Nursing

CHAPTER 35

Psychiatric Consultation-Liaison Nursing

This chapter focuses on the unique role of the psychiatric nurse consultant-liaison. The four phases of the consultation process are addressed, along with the special skills that this nurse specialist must possess in order to function appropriately.

Reading Assignment

Prior to beginning this assignment, please read Chapter 35, "Psychiatric Consultation-Liaison Nursing."

Activities

Using the content in the text, answer the following questions as clearly as you can and in your own words. Give examples, if appropriate, to help clarify the information in your answer.

1. Give examples of each of the areas of psychiatric and general consultation in the advanced-practice psychiatric nurse role. (Table 35–2, pp. 1051–1052)

    a. _____   k. _____

    b. _____   l. _____

    c. _____   m. _____

    d. _____   n. _____

    e. _____   o. _____

    f. _____   p. _____

    g. _____   q. _____

    h. _____   r. _____

    i. _____   s. _____

    j. _____   t. _____

2. Give examples of each area of medical-surgical consultation in the psychiatric nurse practitioner role. (Table 35–2, p. 1051–1052)

a. _____   k. _____
b. _____   l. _____
c. _____   m. _____
d. _____   n. _____
e. _____   o. _____
f. _____   p. _____
g. _____   q. _____
h. _____   r. _____
i. _____   s. _____
j. _____   t. _____

3. Give examples of each area of administrative/employee-related consultation in the advanced-practice psychiatric nurse role. (Table 35–2, p. 1051–1052)

a. _____   k. _____
b. _____   l. _____
c. _____   m. _____
d. _____   n. _____
e. _____   o. _____
f. _____   p. _____
g. _____   q. _____
h. _____   r. _____
i. _____   s. _____
j. _____   t. _____

4. Using Lippitt and Lippitt's consultation model, categorize the roles and corresponding activities. (Table 35–4, p. 1055)

Lippitt and Lippitt's Consultation Model

Role	Activities

5. Identify types of consultation for the *client.* (Table 35–6, pp. 1057–1058)

Types of Consultation: Client

Type	Focus	Purpose	Person or Group Primarily Responsible To	Example

6. Identify types of consultation for the *consultee.* (Table 35–6, pp. 1057–1058)

Types of Consultation: Consultee

Type	Focus	Purpose	Person or Group Primarily Responsible To	Example

7. Identify types of consultation for an *organization or system.* (Table 35–6, p. 1058)

Types of Consultation: Organization/System

Type	Focus	Purpose	Person or Group Primarily Responsible To	Example

8. Compare the reasons for direct and indirect methods of consultation in psychiatric consultation-liaison nursing practice. (Table 35–7, p. 1059)

Indications for Direct versus Indirect Method of Consultation

Direct	Indirect

9. Compare the responsibilities of the consultee with those of the consultant. (Table 35–8, p. 1059)

Responsibilities of Consultee and Consultant

Consultee	Consultant

10. Discuss some of the strategies that may be employed to manage resistance to the consultation process. (p. 1066)

a. _____

b. _____

c. _____

d. _____

e. _____

f. _____

g. _____

h. _____

11. Discuss the qualities that must be developed and maintained by the PCLN in order to be effective. (Table 35–10, p. 1067)

Guidelines for Self-Care Plan

Individual	Environmental

Case Study

Suggested answers for Case Studies are provided in the Answers section at the back of this Study Guide.

Scenario:
An organization has a sharp decrease in client satisfaction documented on discharge surveys. The nurse executive of the organization has decided to use a consultant. Although there is an overall decline, there is no one single explanation for the survey results. Numerous departments and individuals are involved. The situation is known throughout the organization, and pressure to return the level of satisfaction to its previous outstanding rating is essential.

1. Does the situation warrant a direct or indirect method of consultation?

    _____

    _____

    _____

    _____

    _____

2. Why or why not?

    _____

    _____

    _____

    _____

    _____

3. What might the initial activities of the consultant include?

    _____

    _____

    _____

    _____

    _____

Self-Assessment Questions

Answers and rationales for Self-Assessment Questions are provided in the Answers section at the back of this Study Guide.

1. An advanced-practice psychiatric nurse at a large hospital recognizes the area's lack of preparedness should a major disaster occur. Working through channels of communication in the hospital and through local government, the nurse is instrumental in obtaining disaster preparedness grants from the federal government and develops a program. This activity is an example of which type of role?

    a. Entrepreneur

    b. Intrapreneur

    c. Liaison

    d. Consultant

2. An advanced-practice psychiatric nurse plans and initiates his own counseling service. The nurse sees clients individually and provides group therapy for adolescents. The business is so successful that he plans to expand by hiring two additional advanced-practice psychiatric nurses. This is an example of which type of role?

    a. Entrepreneur

    b. Intrapreneur

    c. Liaison

    d. Consultant

3. A school of nursing is planning a major curriculum change. For the psychiatric content, the faculty decides to hire an advanced-practice psychiatric nurse to assist with the outcomes. The role of the hired individual is best described as:

    a. Entrepreneur

    b. Intrapreneur

    c. Liaison

    d. Consultant

4. The oncology unit of a large city hospital has numerous admissions each year. The clients range from those newly diagnosed to those in the terminal stages of disease. The clients and their families are anxious, stressed, and coping with diseases with which they have little if any experience. The staff of the unit is highly competent but is faced with death-related experiences on a daily basis. The unit director has decided to hire someone to meet psychosocial needs of staff, clients, and families. The role this new hire would fill is most likely:

   a. Entrepreneur

   b. Intrapreneur

   c. Liaison

   d. Consultant

5. A small rural hospital has admitted an actively hallucinating client with schizophrenia who is in labor. The birth is imminent. The nurse midwife and the staff are competent and confident in their skills in delivering the baby but are challenged by the active symptoms of the woman's schizophrenia. The most effective approach for this situation is to:

   a. Access telemental health services

   b. Transport the woman to the nearest large hospital, over 200 miles away

   c. Focus on the birth of the baby and consider the mental illness later

   d. Have the woman's family take her to the nearest large hospital, over 200 miles away

6. A nurse on the oncology unit where the staff includes a psychiatric consultation-liaison nurse (PCLN) asks the PCLN about her position. "I had never heard anything before about a position like yours. Is it a new role?" The PCLN's best response is:

   a. "Yes, this type of role is new. There are only one or two nurses in the country."

   b. "No one has heard of PCLN before because there isn't a need for our position except just in a few situations like this."

   c. "Actually no, the PCLN role started over 40 years ago."

   d. "Well, anyone can do it, so I imagine there are lots of us. We just aren't very organized."

7. As a consultant, a nurse collects data and stimulates the thinking of the employees of the organization that has hired the consultant. Which role of Lippitt and Lippitt's model do these activities describe?

   a. Advocate

   b. Alternative identifier

   c. Fact finder

   d. Informational expert

8. As a consultant, a nurse generates options and collaborates with numerous employees throughout the organization that has hired the consultant. Which role of Lippitt and Lippitt's model do these activities describe?

   a. Advocate

   b. Joint problem solver

   c. Objective observer

   d. Trainer

9. A consultant has been asked to meet with a community mental health center to participate in planning for the future. In the course of the work, the consultant identifies the complete purpose of the consultation. Which phase of the consultation process does this describe?

    a. Entry

    b. Diagnosis

    c. Response

    d. Closure/evaluation

10. A consultant has been hired by a community mental health system to review the policies and procedures and to make recommendations to improve the current policies and procedures. This type of consultation is:

    a. Client–direct

    b. Intragroup–indirect

    c. Client–indirect

    d. Organizational–indirect

—NOTES—

CHAPTER 36

Psychiatric Nursing Research

Because there is a paucity of research in psychiatric nursing, this chapter provides an outline for the beginning researcher to follow. Also included is a look at the future of psychiatric nursing research, as well as some of the barriers to psychiatric research.

Reading Assignment

Prior to beginning this assignment, please read Chapter 36, "Psychiatric Nursing Research."

Activities

Using the content in the text, answer the following questions as clearly as you can and in your own words. Give examples, if appropriate, to help clarify the information in your answer.

1. Discuss some potential topics for nursing research. (p. 1076)

    a. _____

    b. _____

    c. _____

    d. _____

    e. _____

    f. _____

    g. _____

    h. _____

    i. _____

    j. _____

2. Give examples of how the following contributing issues in research related to psychiatric–mental health nursing may be addressed. (pp. 1077–1078)

Neurobiological factors_____

_____

_____

Stress and coping _____

_____

_____

Life span issues_____

_____

_____

Psychosocial factors _____

_____

_____

Biobehavioral factors _____

_____

_____

Technological factors _____

_____

_____

3. Identify the 10 steps in the scientific research process, and explain what each step entails. (pp. 1078–1080)

Steps in the Scientific Research Process

Step	Explanation
1.	
2.	
3.	
4.	
5.	
6.	
7.	
8.	
9.	
10.	

4. Describe the role of each of the following in the research process. Give examples of each. (pp. 1080–1083)

The generalist nurse _____

_____

_____

The advanced-practice nurse _____

_____

_____

Principal investigator _____

_____

_____

Member of a research team _____

_____

_____

Data collector _____

_____

_____

Client advocate _____

_____

_____

Critiquer of research findings _____

_____

_____

User of research findings _____

_____

_____

5. Compare the quantitative and qualitative methods of research. (Table 36–4, p. 1086)

Quantitative and Qualitative Research Characteristics

Quantitative Research	Qualitative Research

6. Discuss the 2006–2010 goals of the National Institute of Nursing Research. (p. 1087)

_____

_____

_____

_____

_____

_____

_____

_____

_____

_____

Case Study

Suggested answers for Case Studies are provided in the Answers section at the back of this Study Guide.

Scenario:
A co-worker comes into work and begins to hand out questionnaires to clients on your unit. One of the patients asks you to help complete the information on the form. You notice that the questionnaire asks the client to rate his opinions about mental illness and you can see that it is not a hospital-initiated form. Later you ask the co-worker about the questionnaire. She states that it is a school assignment for a research class.

1. Can the co-worker use the clients on the unit as subjects in a research study?

    _____

    _____

    _____

    _____

2. Why or why not?

    _____

    _____

    _____

    _____

3. What is your responsibility in regard to the distribution of research questionnaires?

    _____

    _____

    _____

    _____

    _____

Self-Assessment Questions

Answers and rationales for Self-Assessment Questions are provided in the Answers section at the back of this Study Guide.

1. A researcher is interested in the experience of an individual with schizophrenia. The type of study most appropriate to this topic is:
    a. Qualitative
    b. Experimental
    c. Ex post facto
    d. Quantitative

2. A researcher has planned a study to determine the frequency and intensity of visual hallucinations in a population of individuals with psychiatric conditions. The type of study that is most appropriate is:
    a. Qualitative
    b. Phenomenology
    c. Ethnography
    d. Quantitative

3. Which of the following is a hypothesis?
    a. Are psychiatric nurses perceived as imparting empathy more than critical care nurses?
    b. The type of nursing specialty has an effect on client perceptions of empathy.
    c. The purpose of this study was to determine client perceptions of nurse-imparted empathy.
    d. This study found no significant difference between nursing specialty and the perceived impartment of empathy.

4. Which of the following is a problem statement?
    a. Are psychiatric nurses perceived as imparting empathy more than critical care nurses?
    b. The type of nursing specialty has an effect on client perceptions of empathy.
    c. The purpose of this study was to determine client perceptions of nurse-imparted empathy.
    d. This study found no significant difference between nursing specialty and the perceived impartment of empathy.

5. In the following hypothesis, what is the independent variable? Nursing students in their senior year engage in more professional activities and study more than do freshman nursing students.
    a. Seniors
    b. Freshmen
    c. Type of nursing student
    d. Professional activities

6. In the following hypothesis, what is the dependent variable? Psychiatric nurses are different from critical care nurses in clients' perceptions of imparting empathy.
   a. Psychiatric nurses
   b. Critical care nurses
   c. Empathy
   d. Client's perceptions

7. A researcher collects data by observing the city's homeless population in their normal activities in the city park and taking copious field notes. This type of data collection is most closely associated with which type of research design?
   a. Quantitative
   b. Experimental
   c. Time series
   d. Qualitative

8. A researcher collects data by asking a randomly selected group of clients with schizophrenia to rate the duration and intensity of their auditory hallucinations. This type of data collection is most closely associated with which type of research design?
   a. Quantitative
   b. Qualitative
   c. Phenomenology
   d. Ethnography

9. List the foci of future psychiatric nursing research. Select all that apply.
   a. Integration of biological and behavioral interfaces
   b. History of psychiatric nursing
   c. Biographies of psychiatric nurse leaders
   d. Adoption and adaptation of new technologies
   e. Development of nursing research investigators
   f. Advancement of health promotion and disease prevention
   g. Elimination of health disparities

10. A new graduate nurse on a psychiatric unit has concerns about the level of lethargy she is noticing in clients who are taking a particular medication. Her best course of action is to:
    a. Access the evidence-based literature regarding the medication
    b. Ask a co-worker for the co-worker's opinion
    c. Continue to give the medication as prescribed
    d. Have another nurse give the medication

The Future of Psychiatric Nursing

In this chapter, the roles of the psychiatric nurse are discussed and the importance of development of leadership skills is emphasized. The chapter concludes with a look at this specialty in terms of its position in the future in all arenas of practice.

Reading Assignment

Prior to beginning this assignment, please read Chapter 37, "The Future of Psychiatric Nursing."

Activities

Using the content in the text, answer the following questions as clearly as you can and in your own words. Give examples, if appropriate, to help clarify the information in your answer.

1. Discuss the role of the psychiatric nurse as a provider of care, as a coordinator of care, and as a member of the profession. Give examples of each. (pp. 1095–1096)

   Provider of care_____

   _____

   _____

   Coordinator of care_____

   _____

   _____

   Member of a profession _____

   _____

   _____

2. How have psychiatric nurses shown leadership in the past? Using the content in the text, give examples to support your answers. (pp. 1096–1097)

_____

_____

_____

_____

_____

3. Describe the concept of "empowerment." Give examples. (p. 1096)

_____

_____

_____

_____

_____

4. How can the psychiatric nurse demonstrate leadership skills? Give examples. (pp. 1096–1097)

a. _____

b. _____

c. _____

d. _____

5. Describe the ways in which technological advances in neurobiology and genetics have affected the specialty of psychiatric–mental health nursing. (p. 1101)

_____

_____

_____

_____

6. Explain how the psychiatric–mental health nurse becomes a consumer advocate. (p. 1103)

_____

_____

_____

_____

_____

7. List Deming's 14 points for total quality management. Give examples of each. (Table 37–1, p. 1104)

   1. _____ 8. _____
   2. _____ 9. _____
   3. _____ 10. _____
   4. _____ 11. _____
   5. _____ 12. _____
   6. _____ 13. _____
   7. _____ 14. _____

8. Discuss the impact of technology on psychiatric–mental health nursing practice related to the following areas. Give examples of each. (pp. 1106–1107)

   a. Health informatics_____
   _____
   _____

   b. Nursing informatics _____
   _____
   _____

   c. Computerized documentation and confidentiality_____
   _____
   _____

   d. Continuity of care and cost-effective health care _____
   _____
   _____

   e. Computer networks _____
   _____
   _____

9. Identify the leading health indicators related to the Healthy People 2010 agenda. Discuss examples in your community related to each. (p. 1108)

   • _____
   • _____
   • _____
   • _____
   • _____
   • _____
   • _____
   • _____
   • _____
   • _____

10. List and explain the four examples of case management used by the psychiatric–mental health nurse. (pp. 1110–1111)

Case Management

Example	Explanation
1.	
2.	
3.	
4.	

11. Discuss the services afforded by telehealth. Give examples of each. (p. 1111)

- _____
- _____
- _____
- _____
- _____
- _____
- _____
- _____
- _____

Case Study

Suggested answers for Case Studies are provided in the Answers section at the back of this Study Guide.

Scenario:
Although the state board of nursing requires that all nurses complete 40 hours of continuing education each renewal period for registered nurses, the psychiatric hospital requires that all registered nurse employees complete at least 80 hours. The hospital provides funding for continuing education and offers many additional programs at no cost to its employees. In addition, the types of continuing education must correspond with the area in which a nurse works.

1. Which of Deming's points for total quality management is evident in this situation?

   _____
   _____
   _____
   _____
   _____

2. How can a manager justify the added expense for a continuing education program?

   _____
   _____
   _____
   _____

Self-Assessment Questions

Answers and rationales for Self-Assessment Questions are provided in the Answers section at the back of this Study Guide.

1. A psychiatric nurse is responsible for a circumscribed group of clients in the community with mental illnesses. The typical workday includes calling clients to assess adherence to medication schedules, assisting with aftercare placement for a client being discharged from the hospital, and following up on a client attending a day treatment program. This nurse's role follows which model of health care delivery?

    a. Primary nursing

    b. Team nursing

    c. Case management

    d. Medical model

2. A psychiatric nurse participates in the development of teaching materials for a community mental health program. The nurse also is active in speaking at community events to promote quality care for the mentally ill. These activities are examples of which role of the psychiatric nurse?

    a. Provider of care

    b. Coordinator of care

    c. Member of the profession

    d. Researcher of care

3. A psychiatric nurse is responsible for a circumscribed group of clients in the community with mental illnesses. The typical workday may include calling clients to check on their medication compliance, assisting with aftercare placement for a client being discharged from the hospital, and following up on a client attending a day treatment program. These activities are examples of which role of the psychiatric nurse?

    a. Provider of care

    b. Member of the profession

    c. Coordinator of care

    d. Researcher of care

4. A psychiatric nurse assesses clients prior to ECT and educates families about the ECT process. These activities are examples of which role of the psychiatric nurse?

    a. Provider of care

    b. Member of the profession

    c. Coordinator of care

    d. Researcher of care

5. Which of the following activities indicates concepts of empowerment?
   a. A teacher focused on getting all psychiatric nursing students to complete a care plan on ineffective coping.
   b. A classroom set up to lecture to a large group of psychiatric nursing students
   c. A requirement that all nursing students successfully complete a computer-assisted instruction vignette on therapeutic communication
   d. Small-group discussion with psychiatric nursing students and faculty to debate the issue of stigma and mental illness

6. A community mental health program has ended an incentive program in which therapists were monetarily rewarded for seeing more clients in less time. The elimination of this practice is supported by which of Deming's 14 points for total quality management?
   a. Create constancy of purpose
   b. Adapt a new philosophy
   c. Award business on price alone
   d. Drive out fear

7. The community mental health program has given one person release time to make the decisions to reorganize the program. Which of Deming's 14 points for total quality management does this practice violate?
   a. Adapt a new philosophy
   b. Cease dependence on inspection
   c. Break down barriers between staff areas
   d. Put everyone to work on transformation

8. A rural hospital that uses an advanced-practice psychiatric nurse consultation service on a routine basis is an example of which of the following?
   a. Health informatics
   b. Nursing informatics
   c. Computerized documentation
   d. Telemedicine

9. Which of the following is a priority area for America: Healthy People 2010?
   a. Promoting mental health by teaching anger management
   b. Hospitalizing homeless individuals with psychiatric conditions
   c. Emphasizing the importance of the handwritten record
   d. Reacting to the surge of new cases of methamphetamine abuse

10. The hospice nurse is working with a family whose father has terminal cancer. During her care, she encourages the family members to talk about death and what death means to each member of the family. She teaches the signs and symptoms of impending death. These interventions are examples of:

    a. Anticipatory guidance

    b. Family therapy

    c. Individual psychotherapy

    d. Behavior therapy

—NOTES—

Answers

Chapter 1: History of Psychiatric Nursing
Case Study

1. The past provides a context to the present.

2. The stigma associated with mental illness that is experienced today has its roots in the misconceptions and treatment of the mentally ill in the eighteenth, nineteenth, and twentieth centuries.

Self-Assessment Questions

1. Answer: a. The focus of care was on a disease medical model rather than on the client.

2. Answer: b. Collaboration on the standards of care was the focus of psychiatric–mental health organizations and the ANA.

3. Answer: d. Psychiatric nurses do not give advice, but they do establish relationships with clients, teach, and assess.

4. Answer: a. In the Middle Ages, the mentally ill were often placed in prisons and treated like criminals. Mesmerism, moral treatment, and humane treatment began in the eighteenth and nineteenth centuries.

5. Answer: a. Psychosexual causes for mental illness were first suggested in the early twentieth century. Neurobiology, neurotransmitters, and brain disease concepts came later in the twentieth century.

6. Answer: a. The nineteenth century saw the founding of the first hospital for the treatment of mental illness.

7. Answer: d. Hildegard Peplau and others stressed the importance of the nurse-client relationship. During the 1700s and 1800s, the focus was on custodial care. During 1920–1940, nursing care was focused on the disease model.

8. Answer: c. The community mental health movement brought changes in the way the mentally ill were treated. Clients were discharged to community-based services.

9. Answer: a. Clients use a variety of complementary therapies and have the right to make those choices. The nurse's role is to support the client. Many complementary therapies do not contradict conventional therapies, although there may be drug-drug interactions.

Chapter 2: Concepts of Psychiatric Care: Therapeutic Models
Case Study

1. Systems theory

2. The client should be treated within the context of the system from which he developed; therefore, family therapy should be considered.

Self-Assessment Questions

1. Answer: c. Teaching is the main focus of cognitive therapy.

2. Answer: c. Dopamine. Serotonin and norepinephrine are associated with depression. GABA is associated with anxiety.

3. Answer: b. Peplau believed that the relationship between client and nurse was therapeutic.

4. Answer: d. Positive reinforcement is a form of behavior therapy.

5. Answer: a. A person who displays direction and purpose has indicated successful fulfillment of Erikson's initiative versus guilt stage of ego development. Trust-mistrust is associated with drive and hope. Autonomy-shame/doubt is associated with self-control and willpower. Intimacy–role confusion is associated with devotion and fidelity.

6. Answer: c. The superego is associated with reward and punishment. The id is associated with the pleasure principle. The ego is associated with the reality principle.

7. Answer: c. Intellectualization has elements of rationalization and magical thinking. The client is using this mechanism to avoid any feeling of responsibility for the loss of his job.

8. Answer: b. Stinginess is associated with the anal stage of psychosexual growth and development.

9. Answer: b. Interpersonal social theory emphasizes the relationship between individuals.

10. Answer: c. Punishment is an aversion event contingent on a response.

Chapter 3: Interfacing Biological-Behavioral Concepts into Psychiatric Nursing Practice
Case Study

1. Genetic

2. Anatomy, physiology, pathophysiology, biology, chemistry

3. Pharmacologic, family therapy

Self-Assessment Questions

1. Answer: c. GABA is associated with anxiety disorders. Dopamine is associated with schizophrenia. Norepinephrine is associated with depression. Acetylcholine is associated with neurodegeneration.

2. Answer: a. Depression is associated with the decreased availability of serotonin, norepinephrine or both.

3. Answer: a. EEG measures electrical activity of the brain. Lesions may be identified by computed tomographic scan. Positron emission tomography is associated with brain functioning, and magnetic resonance imaging is associated with edema, ischemia, infection, or trauma.

4. Answer: a. Serotonin is associated with depression. Dopamine abnormality is most closely associated with schizophrenia.

5. Answer: d. Alzheimer's is associated with brain degeneration. Limbic stimulation is more closely associated with anxiety disorders. Ventricle size is not associated with Alzheimer's. There is no correlation with trauma and the incidence of Alzheimer's.

6. Answer: d. The comparison of incidence of mental illness between monozygotic and dizygotic twins helps to determine whether environment or genetics influence the development an illness.

7. Answer: c. Neurobiological theory focuses on brain function and genetics. A holistic approach integrates environmental, developmental, and genetic influences.

Chapter 4: Foundations of Psychiatric Nursing
Case Study

1. Lies in bed all day, suicidal, rarely bathes, refuses meals, and speaks only when spoken to

2. Withdrawn, quiet, has no friends, socializes with family only

3. Cluster C

4. Diabetes

5. Eviction, low-paying job

6. Living with parents, lack of ADLs

7. Regression

Self-Assessment Questions

1. Answer: a. "Therapeutic use of self" refers to forming a trusting relationship that provides comfort, safety, and acceptance of the client.

2. Answer: b. The diagnosis phase is associated with discerning the need for and purpose of the referral.

3. Answer: c. Irrelevant appraisals take place when the person confronts external occurrences that do not pose a threat to a person's livelihood.

4. Answer: b, f, and g are correct. The client's comments indicate hope, control over the situation, and use of a problem-solving approach.

5. Answer: a. Displacement redirects negative urges to a safer or neutral substitute.

6. Answer: c. The other responses, a, b, and d, are all sympathetic responses and not empathetic.

7. Answer: b. Genuineness is when a person's verbal and nonverbal communication is congruent.

8. Answer: b. Denial is a refusal to admit to a reality, which is treated as though it does not exist.

9. Answer: c. Rationalization is an effort to replace or justify acceptable reasons for a behavior's real reasons.

10. Answer: b. Axis II is associated with personality disorders and mental retardation disorders.

Chapter 5: The Nursing Process
Case Study

1. Sleep pattern disturbance, appetite disturbance, feelings of depression

2. Describe your usual sleeping pattern. What is a typical day of meals for you? Do you have thoughts of killing yourself?

3. Ineffective coping, potential for self-directed violence, social isolation, self-care deficit

Self-Assessment Questions

1. Answer: a. This is an example of testing for recent memory.

2. Answer: c. Abstract reasoning is tested using proverbs.

3. Answer: a. Hyperthyroidism and hypothyroidism can have symptoms similar to some psychiatric symptoms, such as disturbed sleep patterns and energy levels.

4. Answer: b. Spiritual assessment is more than religion. It includes more than organized religious practices.

5. Answer: d. These data indicate that the client's condition is improving.

6. Answer: b. The client's comments indicate there is a problem with problem solving and decision making.

7. Answer: c. Physical harm toward self has a higher priority than the other choices.

8. Answer: a. Hallucinations are a form of disturbance of the senses and perception.

Chapter 6: Therapeutic Communication
Case Study

1. Blocking the only exit and standing over the client

2. Nontherapeutic, because it reinforces the delusion

3. Thought disturbance

4. "I hear that you are very frightened. Professional staff are here for you to talk with at any time about your feelings."

Self-Assessment Questions

1. Answer: c. The nurses' behaviors are barriers to therapeutic communication.

2. Answer: b. Another professional can be supportive to the client. It is important that the needs of others are also met.

3. Answer: a. Only asks the client to reflect on his feelings.

4. Answer: b. Shares the nurse's reality with the client.

5. Answer: b. Instills doubt without arguing with the client.

6. Answer: d. Defending is nontherapeutic.

7. Answer: b. Stating the implied is a therapeutic technique.

8. Answer: b. The client and nurse have mutually identified the problem and begin to work on the issue.

9. Answer: a. Indicates that the nurse is self-monitoring for issues of transference.

10. Answer: a. Indicates that the nurse is trying to see the situation from the client's point of view.

Chapter 7: Cultural and Ethnic Considerations
Case Study

1. Determining the family's beliefs about health and illness

2. Interviewing the client in a language that the client understands, perhaps with an interpreter

3. Setting aside one's own values and beliefs

Self-Assessment Questions

1. Answer: c. Nurses need to be aware of subtle cultural beliefs because the therapeutic relationship can be compromised unknowingly.

2. Answer: a. European Americans as a group are most interested in material goods.

3. Answer: a. The literature indicates that chemical reactions are affected by a person's age, gender, physical size, and genetic patterns in the absorption, distribution, metabolism, and elimination of pharmacologic agents.

4. Answer: d. The stress of African American socioeconomic situations can cause an increase in the incidence of mental illnesses.

5. Answer: d. Asian Americans may need smaller doses of anxiolytics, antidepressants, and lithium than other ethnic groups because Asian Americans metabolize these drugs at a slower rate.

Chapter 8: Legal and Ethical Considerations
Case Study

1. No

2. He has not demonstrated potential for harm to self or others.

3. From the data presented, he does not require hospitalization but should be assessed for medication and follow-up care, likely in an outpatient or community setting.

4. Although he is ill, he is not an immediate danger to self or others. He can be treated in a community or outpatient setting.

5. Depending on the ethical concept, the client should or shouldn't be admitted. If the client wants admission and seeks it, the ethical principle of autonomy may be important. If the hospital is full, with no available beds and other clients who may have more severe symptoms, then he should not be admitted before them. Then justice for the other clients would be important to consider.

Self-Assessment Questions

1. Answer: b. Battery is the unconsented touching of a client. Assault is the threat of touching someone without consent. Slander is when an untruth is stated publicly. Negligence is an unintended outcome of care.

2. Answer: b. The nurse did not allow the client the opportunity to refuse consent.

3. Answer: a. A client's right to informed consent may be waived at the discretion of the nurses and physicians only if a true life-threatening emergency exists.

4. Answer: a. The Fourteenth Amendment is a constitutional right stating that liberty cannot be denied without an impartial hearing. Disability rights are related to protection from discrimination. The right treatment is related to the availability of mental health services. Informed consent is based on the belief that clients should have control over their own bodies.

5. Answer: b. Americans with a mental impairment are qualified to be protected against discrimination in employment. The Fourteenth Amendment is a constitutional right stating that liberty cannot be denied without an impartial hearing. The right to treatment is related to the availability of mental health services. Informed consent is based on the belief that clients should have control over their own bodies.

6. Answer: b. The United States Supreme Court determined that a state cannot be forced to provide treatment where none exists.

7. Answer: d. The nurse must carefully guard the confidentiality of the client's admission. The other responses let the caller know he is an admitted client.

8. Answer: b. The nurse has a duty to the client to give only medications with which the nurse is familiar.

9. Answer: c. The only new right the client has is the right to refuse treatment. The other activities he was able to do even while involuntarily admitted.

10. Answer: d. All are allowed except a co-worker who does not provide direct care to a client.

Chapter 9: The Client with a Depressive Disorder
Case Study

1. Early waking; lost appetite with resulting weight loss, duration of 3 months; loss of interest in activities that were formally enjoyable for him; statements of despair; poor hygiene; sad affect

2. He must be assessed for suicide potential.

3. Potential for violence directed at self

4. Altered nutrition: less than body requirements, self-care deficit, social isolation

5. Antidepressants, suicide precautions, and cognitive, individual, and family therapy

Self-Assessment Questions

1. Answer: a. Antidepressant effects take 2 to 4 weeks.

2. Answer: a. Antidepressants increase serotonin.

3. Answer: d. Choice a is an example of learned helplessness. Choice b. is an example of psychosocial factors. Choice c. is an example of cognitive theory.

4. Answer: a. Choice a acknowledges the client's feelings.

5. Answer: d. All-or-nothing thinking is a form of cognitive distortion.

6. Answer: b. Willpower has no bearing on the outcome of depression. The other statements are factual.

7. Answer: a. Feelings of sadness are less frequent in adolescent depression. Poor school performance and somatic complaints are common characteristics of depression in adolescence.

8. Answer: c. There are five symptoms associated with the diagnostic criteria for major depressive episode. High blood pressure, high white blood cell count, and low heart rate are not symptoms of depression.

9. Answer: c. Dementia has an insidious onset. Forgetfulness is constant, and orientation is impaired with dementia.

10. Answer: d. The client should be in a safe environment to reduce the risk of self-harm. Isolating behaviors are not therapeutic. The nurse should begin teaching at the onset of treatment. The client should be given activities in which she will experience success.

Chapter 10: The Client with a Bipolar Disorder
Case Study

1. Inability to sleep, irritability/labile/hostile behavior, excessive motor ability, delusional, flight of ideas, projection, limited attention span

2. Does he have thoughts of hurting himself or others? When did he last sleep? Is he allergic to any medications? When did he last eat? When did he last use the bathroom? Is he hearing any voices when no one else is around? Is he seeing anything unusual?

3. Risk for other-directed violence

4. Risk for injury, imbalanced nutrition, disturbed thought process, impaired social interactions, disturbed sleep pattern

5. Mood stabilizers, antipsychotics, and short-term benzodiazepines may be used for acute agitation.

Self-Assessment Questions

1. Answer: b. Answer a is most likely bipolar I. Answer c is most likely cyclothymia. Answer d does not have enough information to distinguish between several possible diagnoses.

2. Answer: c. The most recent research indicates that the development of a bipolar disorder is related to neurochemical, neuroendocrine, or neuroanatomical abnormalities. Data support a genetic or biological cause.

3. Answer: a. Children with mania are most likely to be irritable and prone to destructive tantrums rather than overly happy and elated.

4. Answer: d. Lithium can treat active mania and also can prevent future manic episodes. It is not addictive.

5. Answer: d. Impulsive behavior during a manic episode may take the form of harming others.

6. Answer: c. Antipsychotics are used as an adjunct to a mood stabilizer when psychotic features are present. Anticonvulsants are effective in treating bipolar disorder and are often ordered instead of lithium.

7. Answer: a. Even though the client has episodes of depression, an antidepressant is the least likely to be prescribed because of the risk of "switching" a client from a depressive episode to a manic or hypomanic episode. The other medications are often used with bipolar clients.

8. Answer: c. Clients with bipolar disorder should maintain a regular sleep pattern instead of rotating shifts.

9. Answer: d. An invitation to talk more can lead to therapeutic distraction. Although the client may need some medication, this isn't the first choice and may make the client think he is not being heard. Correcting the client's delusion is counterproductive and serves to increase agitation and risk of violence.

10. Answer: c. Sleeping a major portion of the night shows progress for a manic client. Even though the client is eating, it is with prompts. A decrease in the amount of body art is not as significant as the client's being able to sleep. Taking medication does not necessarily indicate improvement.

Chapter 11: The Client with an Anxiety Disorder
Case Study

1. Feeling as though one might die, shortness of breath, elevated heart rate and diaphoresis, confusion, lack of laboratory support for a physical condition

2. Cognitive and individual therapy

3. Signs and symptoms of stress and techniques to decrease stress in one's life; a referral to community mental health services

Self-Assessment Questions

1. Answer: d. Mild anxiety can increase concentration and be conducive to performance. Moderate and severe panic levels of anxiety may produce the other options.

2. Answer: c. Ritualistic behaviors reduce perceived anxiety. There is not enough information to indicate whether the client has feelings of guilt or need for punishment. Although secondary gain may be a part of the dynamics, it is not the primary reason for the behavior.

3. Answer: a. Ritualistic behavior reduces feelings of anxiety.

4. Answer: c. Clients with severe anxiety may unexpectedly threaten or cause harm to self or others.

5. Answer: d. Hypervigilance is associated with acute stress disorder. Hallucinations are associated with psychotic disorders. Motor coordination problems and confusion may be seen in panic disorders.

6. Answer: a. Fear is the primary nursing diagnosis. The other diagnoses may be pertinent but are not of as high a priority.

7. Answer: d. Techniques used to reduce anxiety are effective long term. Long-term use of anxiolytics or hypnotics is inappropriate and may actually worsen anxiety. Electroconvulsive therapy is not appropriate for anxiety disorders.

8. Answer: a. The neurotransmitter affected by anxiolytic medication is GABA.

9. Answer: b. Social phobia is the fear of performance in public. Rituals and trauma are not associated with this phobia. It is unrealistic to avoid all expectations in public.

10. Answer: a. Systematic desensitization is maintaining a state of relaxation while imaging various stages of ranked anxiety-evoking situations.

Chapter 12: The Client with a Somatization Disorder Case Study

1. Conversion disorder

2. Individual psychotherapy using a nonjudgmental, active listening approach

3. Prognosis can be excellent with therapy.

Self-Assessment Questions

1. Answer: a. The primary gain is not feeling the anxiety. Secondary gain is when a client has unintended benefits of the conversion reaction, such as sympathy and gifts of food. Indifference is associated with conversion reaction, but not the primary gain.

2. Answer: b. The client is unable to cope with her feelings of guilt and anxiety.

3. Answer: b. The client is showing insight into the conversion reaction instead of denying or rationalizing her anxiety and symptoms.

4. Answer: d. Depression is considered universal with fibromyalgia clients. The pain is widespread and is located in 11 to 18 tender points. Sleep is often disrupted.

5. Answer: a: The client with hypochondriasis actually experiences the symptoms but exaggerates their seriousness. The symptoms are not hallucinations, and the client is not intentionally faking the symptoms. The symptoms do not warrant or normally respond to medical interventions.

6. Answer: d. The client is aware that there isn't anything seriously wrong with her. The other options indicate that the client still believes there is something wrong.

7. Answer: a. The client is unable to work or interact meaningfully with others. The other diagnoses are not priorities for this client.

8. Answer: c. Body dysmorphic disorder is characterized by a preoccupation with imagined defect in appearance.

9. Answer: b. Malingering is defined as intentionally faking illness for secondary gain. The client is conscious of the behavior.

Chapter 13: The Client with a Stress-Related Disorder
Case Study

1. Cognitive therapy can help the client learn techniques of biofeedback and other stress-reducing activities

2. Ineffective coping

3. Questions should include assessments about family history of heart disease, coping styles, psychosocial stressors, and interpersonal relationships.

Self-Assessment Questions

1. Answer: d. The client will need to follow strict medical regimens and will have enormous emotional needs and intense psychosocial stress.

2. Answer: a. Stress-related disorders are related to unresolved feelings of anxiety, anger, stress or all of these. It is important that clients are first able to recognize feelings before being able to implement techniques to control them.

3. Answer: b. Although there is some controversy, Type A personality has been associated with several stress-related disorders. Internal locus of control, optimism, and problem-solving abilities are successful coping traits.

4. Answer: a. Electronic measurement of a client's psychophysiological responses provides immediate feedback and helps the client to control body responses. Medication is not necessary for biofeedback. Option d describes systematic desensitization.

5. Answer: a. It is important that the client maintain an adequate caloric intake, due to frequent bouts with diarrhea. Fluids can still be absorbed through the stomach. The client is still able to eat. Growth and development may be somewhat affected, but choice a is the highest priority.

6. Answer: a. Clients with coronary heart disease tend to be critical and angry rather than cheerful, funny, or flexible.

7. Answer: b. Asthma is not caused by stress, but stress can exacerbate the symptoms of asthma. There is no support for dependency needs or anger in the cause of asthma.

Chapter 14: The Client with Schizophrenia and Other Psychotic Disorders Case Study

1. Curled up on his bed, withdrawing to the corner of the room

2. Hallucinations, inappropriate laughter, delusions

3. Disorganized behavior, unkempt appearance

4. Disturbed thought patterns, sensory-perceptual disturbance

5. Antipsychotic medications, milieu therapy, group therapy

6. An antipsychotic medication with possibly other medications to counteract the side effects depending on type of antipsychotic prescription

Self-Assessment Questions

1. Answer: d. The other options are examples of positive symptoms of schizophrenia.

2. Answer: b. Echopraxia is a repetition of a behavior that is observed. Echolalia is when a client repeats words he or she hears. Imitation is not a psychotic symptom. Avolition is a marked decrease in motivation.

3. Answer: d. Clang associations are rhymes in a nonsensical pattern. Tangentiality is a symptom in which the client never gets to the point of the conversation. Word salad is a jumble of words. Concrete thinking is when a client has difficulty thinking on the abstract level.

4. Answer: c. Concrete thinking is a response that is literal. Neologisms are invented words. Circumstantiality is when there is a delay in reaching the point of the conversation. Hallucinations are false sensory perceptions.

5. Answer: a. Delusions of grandeur are exaggerated feelings of importance. Delusions of persecution are related to fears of being harmed or persecuted. Delusions of reference are when all events refer specifically to the person. Delusions of control occur when clients believe that others have control over them.

6. Answer: a. The nurse must answer honestly without reinforcing or validating the visual hallucination. Denying that the client is seeing things is counterproductive.

7. Answer: b. Some clients find voice dismissal by exerting conscious control over the voices. Distraction such as being involved in an activity or listening to a radio can help some clients. Touching is not recommended because it can be perceived as threatening by the actively hallucinating client.

8. Answer: a. Catatonia is characterized by stupor, rigid posture, or mutism. Answer b describes paranoid schizophrenia. Answer c is associated with residual schizophrenia. Answer d describes disorganized schizophrenia.

9. Answer: b. The nursing diagnosis for hallucinations is disturbed sensory perception.

10. Answer: c. There is no evidence that stress causes schizophrenia, but it can exacerbate symptoms. Studies have linked genetics, anatomical differences, and dopamine levels with schizophrenia.

Chapter 15: The Client with a Personality Disorder
Case Study

1. Borderline personality disorder

2. Theory of object relations

3. Potential for violence: self-directed

4. Individual and dialectical behavioral therapy

Self-Assessment Questions

1. Answer: a. Schizotypal behavior is associated with peculiar beliefs and appearance, magical thinking, and social isolation. Narcissistic individuals have a grandiose sense of self. Avoidant individuals withdraw because of fear of rejection. Passive-aggressive individuals are obstructionists or procrastinators.

2. Answer: d. Recognizing boundaries is important to delineate with whom and how people interact.

3. Answer: b. Of the symptoms listed, only cruelty to animals is associated with conduct disorders.

4. Answer: a. The prognosis is very poor for conduct disorders. There is some support that temperament is associated with the development of conduct disorders. It is estimated that boys are diagnosed about 9 percent of the time and girls only 2 percent. Truancy is a common characteristic of conduct disorders.

5. Answer: d. Frequent refusal to do chores is a common characteristic of oppositional defiant disorder. The other behaviors are associated with conduct disorder.

6. Answer: a. Antipsychotic medication may be prescribed for Cluster I disorders. The other choices are Cluster II personality disorders.

7. Answer: b. Narcissism has all of these features: a grandiose sense of self-importance, preoccupation with fantasies of success and power, and belief that one is special and should associate only with other special individuals. Histrionic individuals are self-dramatizing. Antisocial individuals lack guilt. Avoidant individuals are fearful of criticism.

8. Answer: a. Acknowledging the client's accomplishments reinforces independent functioning. Offering self, drawing the client into one-on-one interactions, and building trust are important with other personality disorders but not borderline personality disorders.

9. Answer: a. A client who is having trouble with boundaries may think that the nurse can read his mind. Verbalizing feelings and confronting projection can be therapeutic.

10. Answer: d. Choices a, b, and c provide unneeded attention to the wound.

Chapter 16: The Client with Delirium, Dementia, Amnestic, and Other Cognitive Disorders
Case Study

1. Rote and remote memory assessment; thorough physical workup; results of diagnostic and laboratory studies, such as CBC with differential, electrolytes, and so on

2. The mother's safety and the safety of others

3. Alzheimer's has no cure, but there are medications and activities that can slow the progression of the disease

4. Cholinesterase inhibitors, such as Donezepil (Aricept), galanamine (Reminyl), memantine (Namenda)

Self-Assessment Questions

1. Answer: b. Acalculia is the inability to do simple arithmetic. Abulia are functional errors of omission. Anomia is the inability to recall or recognize names of objects. Apraxic agraphia is the inability to express oneself in writing.

2. Answer: c. Anomia is the inability to do simple arithmetic. Abulia are functional errors of omission. Anomia is the inability to recall or recognize names of objects. Apraxia is the inability to carry out familiar movements.

3. Answer: b. Apraxia is the inability to carry out familiar movements, especially the inability to make proper use of an object. Chorea is the ceaseless occurrence of rapid, jerky movements. Delirium is associated with rapid onset. Asimultanagnosia is the inability to visually integrate a complex scene into a coherent whole.

4. Answer: b. Constructional praxis is the inability to copy simple drawings. Apraxic agraphia is the inability to express oneself in writing. Asimultanagnosia is the inability to visually integrate a complex scene into a coherent whole. Semantic paraphasia is substituting a similar word for an object.

5. Answer: b. Choices a, c, and d are associated with dementia.

6. Answer: a. There is no known cure for Alzheimer's. The client will need 24-hour care due to risk of injury, and the family can expect a gradual decline in physical and mental abilities.

7. Answer: a. It is easiest for confused clients to follow simple directions.

8. Answer: c. The client should be in an environment where stimuli are decreased, which includes low lights and few people. Providing reassurance of safety and orienting the client to the surroundings can correct inaccurate perceptions.

9. Answer: d. Although the client did not recently milk his cows, he had done so in the past. This answer reassures the client without lying to him. Choice a is a dishonest answer. Choice b will likely agitate the client further. He can be redirected without the use of medication.

10. Answer: c. The client may not recognize the urge to urinate or move the bowels or may not recognize the bathroom. A routine bladder and bowel schedule that the nursing assistant follows can help to avoid incontinence.

Chapter 17: The Client with Attention-Deficit Disorder
Case Study

1. Onset of symptoms

2. Pharmacologic intervention, family therapy, and behavior contract

3. Psychostimulant such as Adderal

Self-Assessment Questions

1. Answer: c. Attention-deficit/hyperactivity disorder is characterized by distractibility but does not affect appetite or sleep patterns. Repetitive behaviors are seen with obsessive-compulsive disorder.

2. Answer: a. Symptoms must be present before age 7 for a diagnosis of attention deficit with hyperactivity. The other behaviors are not associated with ADHD.

3. Answer: b. Adults do not display the same excessive energy seen but do experience marital difficulties, forgetfulness, and frequent job changes.

4. Answer: b. Choices a, c, and d are common and expected interventions for ADHD. Antipsychotic medication is not appropriate for ADHD.

5. Answer: c. Psychostimulants are the most widely prescribed and best-researched medications used to treat ADHD. The other options are incorrect statements.

6. Answer: a. Psychostimulants are short acting and are effective from 4 to 12 hours. Lab tests are routine evaluations for someone on long-term medication. Psychostimulants have been prescribed for ADHD for approximately 50 years. Medication is started on a low dose and gradually increased until optimal effects are reached.

7. Answer: b. Appetite is most commonly lost with stimulant medication. The other symptoms are common side effects of stimulant medication.

8. Answer: a. The client demonstrates unsuccessful social interaction and an inability to conform to social expectations. There is no evidence for the other choices.

9. Answer: a. This response is respectful of the client without belittling him. Oftentimes clients with ADHD develop low self-esteem, and the teacher's comments should not reinforce this perception.

Chapter 18: The Client with a Dissociative Disorder
Case Study

1. Neurobiology, trauma, stress

2. Individual therapy

3. Active listening, therapeutic communication, cognitive therapy. An advanced-practice psychiatric nurse may be involved in hypnosis.

4. Ineffective coping

Self-Assessment Questions

1. Answer: c. Child abuse is a common experience for individuals diagnosed with dissociative disorder. Although there is some controversy about the existence of the disorder, clients are not faking or manipulating to gain attention.

2. Answer: c. The aim of therapy is to merge all facets of one's personality into a whole. The perception of elimination of an alter will result in resistance to therapy.

3. Answer: a. Fugue is characterized by unexpected travel from home and loss of memory. Malingering is conscious manipulation. Depersonalization is characterized by temporary change in the quality of self-awareness. Dissociative identity disorder is characterized by two or more distinct personalities.

4. Answer: a. Individuals develop fugue in response to intolerable stress by blocking off consciousness.

5. Answer: a. The course of fugue is often brief, lasting hours or days, rarely months. Rarely do clients experience reoccurrences. Psychotherapy is the treatment of choice, rather than pharmacologic interventions. Increased dopamine is associated with schizophrenic disorders.

Chapter 19: The Client at Risk of Suicidal and Self-Destructive Behaviors

Case Study

1. Suicide potential

2. Losses, stressors, lack of support, lethal and available means of committing suicide, older age

3. Potential for violence: self-directed

4. Suicide precautions

Self-Assessment Questions

1. Answer: c. Asking the client about current suicidal potential in a direct manner allows the client to verbalize feelings about suicide and assesses safety. Avoiding the subject, distraction, and focusing on a future event will not keep the client safe.

2. Answer: a. The client may display improvement in affect prior to committing suicide. The nurse should continue suicidal precautions. The other options may give the client a greater opportunity to act upon his suicidal ideation.

3. Answer: b. Men commit suicide in higher numbers than women. Alcoholism is a risk factor.

4. Answer: c. The client may be determining when he will have an opportunity to act on his suicidal ideation.

5. Answer: a. A verbal contract that documents that the client will not harm himself is a specific goal for a suicidal client. Anger is not always associated with suicide. Even though the client may not talk about his suicidal ideation, there may still be ideation about suicide. Seeking out staff to talk about feelings is an important goal but not the highest priority.

6. Answer: a. This option has the highest lethality, and the client has immediate access. The other plans are either more vague or not as accessible.

7. Answer: a. A direct question is the best assessment for suicide. Often clients are relieved to talk about their thoughts. It is a myth that asking about suicide puts the idea into the head of a client.

8. Answer: b. Personality traits such as impulsivity may constitute a temperamental vulnerability to suicide, especially in the presence of maladaptive behavior, as seen in borderline personality disorder.

9. Answer: d. Thoughts of suicide are not normal behavior. The daughter needs a professional evaluation as soon as possible.

10. Answer: c. This response further explores the client's statement to understand the meaning of his comments. The other options either dismiss his concerns or delay the opportunity to assess.

Chapter 20: The Client Exhibiting Aggression, Hostility, and Violence Case Study

1. Acknowledge his feelings

2. Initiate backup support procedures and assess the other clients on the unit

3. Frustration, loss of control, biochemical or neurophysiological reasons

4. Verb de-escalation, active listening, ensuring easy access to staff support in the event of increased escalation

Self-Assessment Questions

1. Answer: a. "Acting out" refers to living out unresolved developmental issues or fantasies impulsively in behavior.

2. Answer: a. This choice allows the client to retain control of his situation, yet limits his options. Challenging the client or daring the client will escalate the situation.

3. Answer: b. Documenting that the client was responsible for the consequences of his behavior affords the nurse some protection from assault and battery. The other choices leave it open to interpretation whether the client's rights were violated.

4. Answer: c. There is evidence for genetic influences for aggression and disruptive behaviors associated with some psychiatric disorders. Judgmental comments, such as "lack of discipline" are discouraged. It is imperative to educate staff about nontherapeutic comments concerning behavioral problems in children and adolescents.

5. Answer: c. Although offering classes is laudable, employees do not have to take advantage of the courses, and some employees may be physically incapable of defending themselves. Violence prevention training should be mandated through policy and documented at least annually. Workplace safety strategies that include activating professional teams to assist with a potential or violent situation are very effective.

6. Answer: d. Unrestricted movement of the public increases the risk of workplace violence. Other factors include working alone and inadequate security staff.

7. Answer: a. Use of blame or displacement is a risk factor. Being able to verbalize feelings, having a stable work history, and not being bullied are not associated with violence.

8. Answer: a. This response seeks to ensure personal dignity, shows respect, is direct and supportive, and establishes a therapeutic relationship.

Chapter 21: The Client with a Substance-Related Disorder
Case Study

1. A complete physical examination, including liver function tests, nutritional status, and skin assessment

2. Issues of dysfunctional communication and relationship patterns

3. Several theories are associated with substance-related disorder. It is primarily a chronic, recurrent disease with neurobiological, genetic, and environmental underpinnings that influence its occurrence and maintenance.

4. It has profound effects on interpersonal relationships in the family system.

Self-Assessment Questions

1. Answer: c. Tolerance is a pharmacologic property of some substances, in which increased amounts over time are required to achieve similar results as in earlier use.

2. Answer: a. This client is showing signs of alcohol withdrawal.

3. Answer: c. Alcohol withdrawal can be a life-threatening situation. The client needs to be evaluated and treated immediately. Although he may need an alcohol evaluation, it is not the priority at this time.

4. Answer: b. An anxiolytic agent is given to prevent and treat delirium tremens. Parenteral route is important because without immediate intervention, the client could develop hyperthermia or cardiovascular collapse or die.

5. Answer: d. Choices a, b, and c are typical questions to assess sensory perceptual disturbances (tactile, auditory, and visual). Liver involvement is not determined by pain in the upper right quadrant.

6. Answer: b. There is little evidence that pain management as part of a medical hospitalization will cause drug dependence. There is support that managing pain with narcotics will not worsen a preexisting drug dependency. Clients heal more effectively when pain is managed.

7. Answer: c. Cola has large amounts of caffeine that can cause sleep disturbances. Running is a healthy activity, and he is doing it early enough in the day to not have it interfere with sleep. An occasional nap will not interfere with sleep on a routine basis. The client appears to have a routine sleep schedule.

8. Answer: a. This comment indicates that the client admits that he is powerless to avoid alcohol and that his life has become unmanageable. Choice b is Step 8. Choice c is Step 5. Choice d is Step 10.

9. Answer: a. Abstinence is the goal of treatment. This statement indicates that the client is already rationalizing. Recovering alcoholic individuals will need the support of a sponsor and will likely need to attend support groups on a frequent basis. Alcoholics Anonymous does not require adherence to all steps of the program but does ask individuals to keep an open mind in the role that the steps can play in a recovery program.

10. Answer: a. Although all of the nursing diagnoses are associated with substance abuse, this client is in immediate danger of injury due to alcohol withdrawal.

Chapter 22: The Client with an Eating Disorder
Case Study

1. Routine laboratory and diagnostic studies, including chemistry profile, electrolytes, cardiovascular studies, thyroid function test

2. Family theorists view interaction within the family system as discouraging the development of independence and autonomy.

3. Medical stabilization/management of caloric, nutritional, and other physical complications caused by eating disorder; psychiatric treatment to include individual and group therapy

Self-Assessment Questions

1. Answer: a. Individuals who routinely vomit to control weight may have pitted enamel from hydrochloric acid in the vomitus.

2. Answer: d. "Body image disturbance" refers to a distortion in the image of the boy that is of near or actual delusional proportions.

3. Answer: b. The student's signs and symptoms are all physiological findings of anorexia nervosa.

4. Answer: d. Bulimia is a habit of eating large amounts followed by purging. Disappearing after meals is likely to involve self-induced vomiting.

5. Answer: c. Vomiting is not associated with pica.

6. Answer: b. Persons in occupations that stress appearance and weight management as a mark of achievement, such as gymnasts, are at high risk.

7. Answer: Choices a, b, e, and h are all common findings upon physiological assessment.

8. Answer: 14.89 $\dfrac{36.8 \text{ kg}}{(1.57 \text{ m})^2} = \dfrac{36.8 \text{ kg}}{2.47 \text{ m}} = 14.89$

9. Answer: a. Her intake of nutrients is insufficient to meet metabolic needs.

10. Answer: a. The client is at high risk for complication. She must eat or be forced to take in nutrients. The other options are also a part of the nursing interventions but do not have a higher priority than the client's consumption of calories.

Chapter 23: The Client with a Sleep Disorder
Case Study

1. Normal eating and sleep habits; substance use, including alcohol and caffeine intake, prescribed and over-the-counter medications, and herbal preparations; recent stressors

2. Sleep hygiene; establish a normal sleep routine; cognitive behavioral therapies

3. Sleep pattern disturbance: more than body requirement

Self-Assessment Questions

1. Answer: d. Stage IV is the stage of sleep in which growth hormone is released.

2. Answer: b. Chocolate has a stimulant that is causing her sleep disturbance. The other activities should not interfere with sleep.

3. Answer: a. All are examples of good sleep hygiene except lying awake in bed. If sleep does not occur after lying awake for 15 minutes, an individual should get out of bed and do something to facilitate sleep, like read.

4. Answer: d. Sleepwalking is characterized by the performance of motor activity initiated during sleep, in which the individual may leave the bed and walk about. Most often the person returns to bed and has no memory of the event on awakening.

5. Answer: b. Asking the client to describe his routine will focus on his current situation. The other questions are not relevant to the current complaints of fatigue.

6. Answer: b. A symptom of depression is early awakening without the ability to fall back to sleep.

7. Answer: a. Eating a high-carbohydrate snack before bedtime can increase the levels of the amino acid tryptophan, a precursor to the neurotransmitter serotonin. Serotonin is thought to play a role in the promotion of sleep. The other activities are known to disrupt sleep.

Chapter 24: The Client with a Sexual Disorder
Case Study

1. The wife should have a comprehensive medical workup, including routine diagnostic and laboratory studies.

2. Depression

3. Neurotransmitter imbalance, genetic predisposition

4. Marital therapy, stress management

Self-Assessment Questions

1. Answer: a. Cardiovascular disease does not require abstinence from sex. The client will need education on when and how to resume relations with his spouse according to his activity tolerance.

2. Answer: c. Children are often uncertain how to bring up sexual issues with parents. Parents have to be open to considering any question appropriate, and the issues need to be addressed at different times and not in one discussion.

3. Answer: c. Acknowledging the client's dilemma allows the nurse to follow up with options that satisfy the client's desire for improvement with his depression and his ability to perform sexually. The other options deny the importance of his sexual activity.

4. Answer: c. Nursing home residents who are able to make decisions on their own behalf have the right to privacy with a family member. Sexual activity may decline somewhat in old age, but many people remain sexually active into their 80s and 90s.

5. Answer: a. Marijuana usage can interfere with sexual physiological response. Although stress and interpersonal relationships can contribute to the sexual dysfunction in this situation, they are not as significant as the marijuana usage.

6. Answer: c. Venlafaxine XR is a selective norepinephrine reuptake inhibitor (SNRI) and like selective serotonin reuptake inhibitors (SSRIs) causes sexual disturbances. Bupropion is also an antidepressant but has fewer sexual side effects than novel antidepressants and is often used as adjunct to reduce sexual side effects.

7. Answer: a. In 1974 the APA voted that homosexuality was not a mental disorder.

Chapter 25: The Client Who Survives Violence
Case Study

1. Assessing clients' physical and psychosocial needs and level of empathy and quality of support from family members and remaining nonjudgmental

2. Family therapy, psychoeducation about stress responses, individual therapy for adolescents

Self-Assessment Questions

1. Answer: a. Bruises in various stages of healing can be a sign of child abuse.

2. Answer: b. The client needs to be interviewed alone to best elicit honest answers. If the daughter is the abuser, the client may not freely answer the nurse's questions.

3. Answer: a. Health care workers are required to report suspected abuse.

4. Answer: c. Acknowledging the daughter's situation can allow the daughter to express her concerns. The focus is not to place blame but to seek the best solution for all.

5. Answer: d. The client's safety is paramount. The nurse needs to establish a rapport and begin to collect data to best help this client.

6. Answer: Choices a, c, and e are clinical signs of shaken baby syndrome.

7. Answer: a. One of the most dangerous times for a battered spouse is when the battered spouse leaves.

8. Answer: b. The behaviors the client is displaying are signs of sexual abuse in the home.

9. Answer: a. Intimate partner violence can be psychological as well as physical. All the other statements are true.

10. Answer: d. Controlling behavior can be associated with intimate partner violence.

Chapter 26: Individual Psychotherapy
Case Study

1. The goal is to use the nurse-client relationship to facilitate adaptive behavioral changes and effective coping responses and promote optimal health.

2. Countertransference issues

3. Use individual psychotherapy using cognitive behavioral techniques to resolve thoughts, feelings, and behaviors that contribute to depression and anxiety.

Self-Assessment Questions

1. Answer: d. Allowing the client to discuss issues of the client's choosing is a form of free association.

2. Answer: b. Countertransference is when the therapist reacts to the client based on the standpoint of therapist's early childhood experiences.

3. Answer: a, b, c, d, e, f, g. All are goals for psychotherapy.

4. Answer: c. Flooding is a type of therapy in which the client experiences that with which the client is phobic.

5. Answer: a. Play therapy is beneficial with young clients because they may not have the language skills to speak about their needs.

6. Answer: d. Therapists cannot promise what they cannot do. If a client admits to behaviors that are criminal or dangerous, the therapist is obligated to report the behaviors.

Chapter 27: Group Therapy
Case Study

1. Instillation of hope

2. Universality

3. Group cohesiveness

Self-Assessment Questions

1. Answer: a. The male client is speaking the way he likely speaks in other male-female relationships.

2. Answer: a. The group therapist's role is to engage the group in the process and not to do individual therapy with an audience.

3. Answer: b. Universality is when problems, thoughts, and feelings are shared by other group members.

4. Answer: b. The group is feeling connected, although on negative feedback.

5. Answer: b. A group with members who share a similar situation is a self-help group.

6. Answer: a. Psychoeducational is the best answer because if clients are inpatients, then emotional issues about their medications are likely. The group will be about more than just how to take medications.

7. Answer: d. The client's active symptoms interfere with his concentration and the thought processes necessary to participate in this activity.

8. Answer: d. Careful selection of the room is important. The group members should feel assured that the conversation is uninterrupted.

9. Answer: c. The minimum preparation for a group therapist is a master's degree with supervised practice.

10. Answer: b. The nurse is responsible to engage the group members in the process.

Chapter 28: Familial Systems and Family Therapy
Case Study

1. Double-bind communication

2. Using the behavioral, biological, and social sciences as the basis, the nurse therapist assesses, identifies family outcomes, and develops interventions to address maladaptive familial interactions and imparted communication patterns.

Self-Assessment Questions

1. Answer: b. The boundary of with whom and how members in a family participate in a relationship has been crossed by the father.

2. Answer: d. Marital schism is when a parent attempts to enlist a child as an ally against the other parent.

3. Answer: b. Marital skew is severe marital discord arising from acceptance of maladaptive behaviors in one partner by the other partner.

4. Answer: b. Scapegoating is a form of displacement that involves blaming a member for the actions of others.

5. Answer: a, b, c, d, and e. Families are defined in multiple ways.

6. Answer: d. Placement into society has not been fully accomplished. Although the son is employed, he does not live independently.

7. Answer: b. "Triangulation" is a term that describes a maladaptive triad, in this case, an attempt to enlist another to agree with a position.

8. Answer: d. Establishing new family traditions and rituals is a major task of blended families.

9. Answer: c. "Relational resilience" refers to the family's ability to mobilize resources and confront stressors.

Chapter 29: Psychopharmacologic Therapy
Case Study

1. Lithium level, electrolytes

2. It is high and near toxic levels.

3. It could be true. He is likely dehydrated because of excessive sodium loss caused by sweating during the race. Sodium loss increases lithium reabsorption and subsequent lithium toxicity.

4. The client needs to learn more about the role of fluids and electrolytes in conjunction with his lithium medication.

Self-Assessment Questions

1. Answer: b. Bananas, especially ripe ones, have tyramine. Tyramine can cause hypertensive crisis in clients taking MOAIs.

2. Answer: c. The client likely has priapism and needs immediate medical intervention. Untreated, impotence can result.

3. Answer: b. Dry mouth is a common side effect of antidepressants. Offering gum, ice, candy, or frequent sips of water can alleviate the symptom.

4. Answer: a. A headache and nausea are symptoms of hypertensive crisis, a severe side effect of MOAIs.

5. Answer: b. Orthostatic hypotension is a common side effect of many antipsychotic agents. The client's blood pressure should be taken lying and standing to determine whether this is occurring. The client should be taught to rise slowly from sitting or lying position.

6. Answer: d. Tongue movements indicate early signs of a serious, potentially irreversible side effect, tardive dyskinesia.

7. Answer: b. The client is showing extrapyramidal symptoms, which are likely a side effect of his antipsychotic medication. Cogentin or another antiparkinsonian agent should be administered should it be ordered.

8. Answer: a. The client's symptoms are consistent with discontinuation syndrome, in which the client abruptly discontinues the prescribed medication and withdrawal symptoms ensue.

9. Answer: a. Uncontrolled rolling back of the eyes is a sign of oculogyric crisis associated with acute dystonia and should be treated as an emergency.

10. Answer: b. The blood level is dangerously high and associated with lithium toxicity, a life-threatening complication.

Chapter 30: Electroconvulsive, Other Biological (Somatic), and Complementary Therapies
Case Study

1. The teaching plan should include elements of the causative factors of seasonal affective disorder and the rationale for using light therapy. Discuss other treatment options, such as antidepressant medication, when indicated.

2. The client's depression should be reevaluated at 7 days and routinely after that.

3. Circadian rhythm is influenced by the light. How decreased sunlight during winter months results in increased melatonin levels associated with seasonal affective disorder.

Self-Assessment Questions

1. Answer: a. Although the exact neurobiological effect of seizures remains unknown, studies indicate changes in neurochemical, neurophysiological, and neuroendocrine processes. Response a is truthful without overcomplicated information and does not belittle the client for asking.

2. Answer: c. The elderly with depression who cannot tolerate traditional antidepressant therapies are good candidates for ECT.

3. Answer: c. The client may experience some confusion immediately after the treatment, but long-term memory remains intact.

4. Answer. a. The goal of the nurse should be to reduce the client's anxiety about the pending procedure. It is unnecessary for the client to have permission from family members. Clients must give permission, but they do not have to be forced to state that it is their preferred treatment option.

5. Answer: a. Studies have indicated that aromatherapy is a unique form of herbal medicine that uses the healing properties of oils.

6. Answer. a. Shift workers whose schedules change have constant variation in the sleep-wake cycle determined by the day-night cycle.

7. Answer: a. ECT was first used as early as 1938 by Italian physicians Ugo Cerletti and Lusiano Bini.

Chapter 31: Crisis Intervention Management: The Role of Adaptation Case Study

1. Primary

2. Demanding or challenging stress

3. Developing adaptive coping mechanisms

Self-Assessment Questions

1. Answer: d. Crisis intervention is short-term, here-and-now focused intervention. The other options are more likely to be long term in nature.

2. Answer: b. The pregnancy has caused the family to communicate in ways that they may not have done before, thus creating new coping mechanisms. The statement by the family is likely a true statement.

3. Answer: d. Intimacy vs. isolation is the task of forming intense interpersonal relationships

4. Answer: d. Accepting assistance is responding in an adaptive manner. The three conditions necessary for crisis are: occurrence of a hazardous event that poses a threat, emotional need, and inability to respond adaptively.

5. Answer: d. Death of a loved one is an interpersonal or psychosocial type of situational crisis. Fires are environmental, riots are environmental, and amputations are physical.

6. Answer: a. Generativity is concerned with establishing, guiding, and contributing to the next generation. Getting married is an example of forming a close meaningful relationship associated with intimacy. Choosing a profession is associated with identity. Following social norms is a part of knowing right from wrong in the initiative vs. guilt stage.

7. Answer: d. Struggle for significance refers to efforts to make sense of almost dying and then surviving a traumatic experience. Death anxiety consists of vivid images of the event. Death guilt relates to having trouble forgiving oneself for surviving. Psychic numbing refers to an impaired capacity to feel.

8. Answer: c. The client is having difficulty adapting to life without her partner. There may be ineffective home maintenance if she is not caring for herself, but there are no data in the question to support that. There may be fear that she might die too, but there are no data in the question to support that. There have been no changes in her body image.

9. Answer: b. Adapting to an environmental event is a form of situational crisis.

10. Answer: a. The goal for the client is to return to at least the previous level of coping before the crisis event. The crisis also gives the client an opportunity to learn new coping skills to achieve an even higher level of functioning.

Chapter 32: Milieu Therapy/Hospital-Based Care
Case Study

1. Structure and more safety, stabilization, and socialization

2. Safety and medication stabilization

Self-Assessment Questions

1. Answer: d. Although all of the elements are therapeutic for the client, in the case of suicide, the reason for the hospitalization is to provide protection for the client.

2. Answer: b. Orienting clients to the schedule of the day and providing the services of the unit is an element of structure.

3. Answer: d. Designing the environment in such a way as to reduce the risk of a successful suicide attempt uses milieu therapy as an intervention for risk for violence directed at self.

4. Answer: c. Although some individuals may see the use of seclusion rooms as punishment and an issue of authority, the careful use of seclusion is based on making use of the environment to structure safety for all.

5. Answer: a. Interactions with others can help shape behavior, especially in children and adolescents.

6. Answer: c. This choice lays the foundation for the nurse-client relationship and is respectful of the client's anxiety.

Chapter 33: Home- and Community-Based Care
Case Study

1. Tertiary

Self-Assessment Questions

1. Answer: a. Early detection can reduce disability and influence prognosis.

2. Answer. d. The case manager may assist in arranging transportation for consumers, but it is inappropriate for case managers to drive clients for nonemergency purposes.

3. Answer: a. Primary prevention includes strategies that reduce a person's risk to develop a mental illness.

4. Answer: b. Secondary prevention involves nurses' use of interventions to reduce the progression of mental illness; in this case, grieving.

5. Answer: c. A day treatment program works well for those clients who need more than traditional outpatient care but less than 24-hour-a-day care.

6. Answer: a, b, c, and e. Community mental health centers provide all of these. The safety of a suicidal client cannot routinely be ensured at a community mental health center.

Chapter 34: Psychosocial Care in Medical-Surgical Settings
Case Study

1. Denial

2. Anger

3. Acknowledge his willingness to help his father

Self-Assessment Questions

1. Answer: a. Acknowledging the client's feeling de-escalates the situation, especially if the nurse keeps her own emotions in check. Patronizing, taking it personally, and discounting a client's feeling can escalate the situation.

2. Answer: a. Touching a client invades the client's space, can be threatening to the client, and can make the client feel cornered.

3. Answer: c. Limiting complaints can interfere with the client gaining insight into his or her feelings.

4. Answer: d. An initial reaction to grief is disbelief.

5. Answer: d. The husband is participating in his wife's care and is prepared for her death.

Chapter 35: Psychiatric Consultation-Liaison Nursing
Case Study

1. Direct

2. The situation is complex, unclear, and convoluted. The consultee is under great pressure.

3. Gather data

Self-Assessment Questions

1. Answer: b. An intrapreneur is an individual who expands the traditional role as a direct health care provider to that of a creator of services.

2. Answer: a. An entrepreneur is an individual who organizes, manages, and risks assumptions of a business venture or enterprise.

3. Answer: d. A consultant is an expert who renders an opinion in response to a request.

4. Answer: c. Liaison is the facilitation of the relationships between the client, the client's illness, the consultee, the health care team, and the environment.

5. Answer: a. Telemental health may be effectively used to replace face-to-face consultation with nurses and other providers, particularly those working in remote or rural practice settings. Transporting the client has the risk of the baby being born en route. Focusing only on the birth would not meet the woman's holistic needs.

6. Answer: c. PCLN role emerged in the 1960s and has a formal and organized structure.

7. Answer: c. The fact-finding role is one in which a consultant collects data, stimulates thinking, and provides information requested.

8. Answer: b. The role of a joint problem solver involves identifying options and alternatives and collaborating with a consultee, team, or both to solve problems.

9. Answer: b. The diagnosis phase of the consultation process is the determination of the need for and purpose of the consultation.

10. Answer: d. Organizational-indirect type of consultation is where the consultant assists administrators and managers to develop proactive processes.

Chapter 36: Psychiatric Nursing Research
Case Study

1. Not without explicit Institutional Review Board approval and the facility's express permission. Then, each client or guardian must give informed consent to participate.

2. The client's ethical rights must be protected.

3. You must stop your co-worker from gathering any data until all approvals and consents are ensured.

Self-Assessment Questions

1. Answer: a. Qualitative research focuses on the meaning of the experience to individuals rather than on the generalizability of study results.

2. Answer: a. Quantitative research focuses on gathering numerical data, with the intent of generalizing the findings of the study.

3. Answer: b. A hypothesis is a prediction about the study results.

4. Answer: c. A problem statement is a narrowed focus statement.

5. Answer: c. The independent variable is the presumed cause. In this hypothesis, staying in college is having an effect on professional activities and studying.

6. Answer: d. The dependent variable is the presumed effect. In this hypothesis, the type of specialty nurse has an effect on client perception.

7. Answer: d. Qualitative designs are focused on holism.

8. Answer: a. Quantitative designs are focused on specific concepts and gathering of numerical data.

9. Answer: a, d, e, f, and g. The strategic plan of the National Institute of Nursing Research does not include historical or biographical foci for the future of nursing research.

10. Answer: a. All nurses are expected to be consumers of research. Decision in practice should be based on scientific inquiry to best meet clients' needs.

Chapter 37: The Future of Psychiatric Nursing
Case Study

1. Education and reeducation is essential.

2. Quality is cost-effective.

Self-Assessment Questions

1. Answer: c. Case management is comprehensive and holistic health care delivery that concentrates the responsibility for all care given to a client in one person or agency.

2. Answer: c. The member-of-the-profession role includes investing time and energy in activities that promote the preservation of psychiatric nursing as well as resources for clients and their families.

3. Answer: c. The coordinator-of-care role includes being a member of an interdisciplinary team or manager of the care of a group of clients.

4. Answer: a. The provider-of-care role is involved in primary care and preventive services.

5. Answer: c. Enpowerment in educational practices means to emphasize learning rather than teaching.

6. Answer: c. Quality of work will be compromised if money is the only consideration.

7. Answer: d. For change that will be accepted and truly transforms an organization, everyone needs to be involved in the process instead of one person making the decisions.

8. Answer: b. "Nursing informatics" refers to the use of technology to meet client health care needs in nontraditional settings.

9. Answer: a. Healthy People 2010 has seven priority areas. These include health promotion, health protection, prevention, data system, age-related objectives, special populations, and goals. The other choices are reactive or outdated activities.

10. Answer: a. Anticipatory guidance is a form of psychoeducation and is the method the professional nurse uses to reduce the risk of disorders in vulnerable populations. This family is at risk for dysfunctional grieving, and by preparing the family for the inevitable death, the nurse is reducing the risk for maladaptive responses.

—NOTES—

—NOTES—

—NOTES—

—NOTES—

—NOTES—